Thyroid and Parathyroid Disease

Editors

AMY Y. CHEN
MICHAEL C. SINGER

OTOLARYNGOLOGIC CLINICS OF NORTH AMERICA

www.oto.theclinics.com

Consulting Editor
SUJANA S. CHANDRASEKHAR

February 2024 • Volume 57 • Number 1

ELSEVIER

1600 John F. Kennedy Boulevard • Suite 1800 • Philadelphia, Pennsylvania, 19103-2899

http://www.oto.theclinics.com

OTOLARYNGOLOGIC CLINICS OF NORTH AMERICA Volume 57, Number 1
February 2024 ISSN 0030-6665, ISBN-13: 978-0-443-24628-9

Editor: Stacy Eastman
Developmental Editor: Malvika Shah

Otolaryngologic Clinics of North America (ISSN 0030-6665) is published bimonthly by Elsevier, Inc., 360 Park Avenue South, New York, NY 10010-1710. Months of issue are February, April, June, August, October, and December. Business and Editorial Offices: 1600 John F. Kennedy Blvd., Suite 1800, Philadelphia, PA 19103-2899. Customer Service Office: 6277 Sea Harbor Drive, Orlando, FL 32887-4800. Periodicals postage paid at New York, NY and additional mailing offices. Subscription prices are $478.00 per year (US individuals), $100.00 per year (US & Canadian student/resident), $623.00 per year (Canadian individuals), $679.00 per year (international individuals), $270.00 per year (international student/resident). For institutional access pricing please contact Customer Service via the contact information below. Foreign air speed delivery is included in all *Clinics*' subscription prices. All prices are subject to change without notice. **POSTMASTER:** Send address changes to *Otolaryngologic Clinics of North America*, Elsevier Health Sciences Division, Subscription Customer Service, 3251 Riverport Lane, Maryland Heights, MO 63043. **Telephone: 1-800-654-2452 (U.S. and Canada); 314-447-8871 (outside U.S. and Canada). Fax: 314-447-8029. E-mail: journalscustomerservice-usa@elsevier.com (for print support); journalsonlinesupport-usa@elsevier.com (for online support).**

Reprints. For copies of 100 or more of articles in this publication, please contact the Commercial Reprints Department, Elsevier Inc., 360 Park Avenue South, New York, NY 10010-1710. Tel.: 212-633-3874; Fax: 212-633-3820; E-mail: reprints@elsevier.com.

Otolaryngologic Clinics of North America is also published in Spanish by McGraw-Hill Interamericana Editores S.A., P.O. Box 5-237, 06500 Mexico D.F., Mexico.

Otolaryngologic Clinics of North America is covered in *MEDLINE/PubMed (Index Medicus), Current Contents/Clinical Medicine, Excerpta Medica, BIOSIS, Science Citation Index,* and *ISI/BIOMED.*

Contributors

CONSULTING EDITOR

SUJANA S. CHANDRASEKHAR, MD, FAAO-HNS, FAOS, FACS
Consulting Editor, *Otolaryngologic Clinics of North America*, President, American Otological Society, Past President, American Academy of Otolaryngology- Head and Neck Surgery, Partner, ENT and Allergy Associates, LLP, Clinical Professor, Department of Otolaryngology–Head and Neck Surgery, Zucker School of Medicine at Hofstra/Northwell, Clinical Associate Professor, Department of Otolaryngology–Head and Neck Surgery, Icahn School of Medicine at Mount Sinai, New York, New York, USA

EDITORS

AMY Y. CHEN, MD, MPH, MBA, FACS
Professor and Vice Chair, Director, Endocrine Surgery, Department of Otolaryngology–Head and Neck Surgery, Emory University, Atlanta, Georgia, USA

MICHAEL C. SINGER, MD, FACS, FACE
Director, Division of Thyroid and Parathyroid Surgery, Department of Otolaryngology–Head and Neck Surgery, Henry Ford Hospital, Detroit, Michigan, USA

AUTHORS

AMR H. ABDELHAMID AHMED, MBBCH, MMSc
Division of Thyroid and Parathyroid Endocrine Surgery, Department of Otolaryngology–Head and Neck Surgery, Massachusetts Eye and Ear Infirmary, Harvard Medical School, Boston, Massachusetts, USA

AMANDA J. BASTIEN, MD
Resident Physician, Division of Otolaryngology–Head and Neck Surgery, Department of Surgery, Samuel Oschin Comprehensive Cancer Institute, Cedars-Sinai Medical Center, Los Angeles, California, USA

CATHERINE ALESSANDRA COLAIANNI, MD, MPhil
Assistant Professor, Otolaryngology–Head and Neck Surgery, Oregon Health and Science University

ELIZABETH E. COTTRILL, MD
Associate Professor, Department of Otolaryngology–Head and Neck Surgery, Thomas Jefferson University Hospital, Philadelphia, Pennsylvania, USA

KAITLYN M. FRAZIER, MD
Resident Physician, Department of Otolaryngology–Head and Neck Surgery, Johns Hopkins School of Medicine, Baltimore, Maryland, USA

ZOE H. FULLERTON, MD, MBE
Resident, Department of Otolaryngology–Head and Neck Surgery, Stanford University, Stanford, California, USA

DAVID GOLDENBERG, MD, FACS
Professor and Chair, Penn State Health Department of Otolaryngology–Head and Neck Surgery, Penn State College of Medicine, Hershey, Pennsylvania, USA

DANA HARTL, MD
Department of Surgery, Thyroid Surgery Unit, Gustave Roussy Cancer Campus, University Paris-Saclay, Paris, France

ALLEN S. HO, MD
Professor, Division of Otolaryngology–Head and Neck Surgery, Department of Surgery, Director, Head and Neck Cancer Program, Samuel Oschin Comprehensive Cancer Institute, Cedars-Sinai Medical Center, Los Angeles, California, USA

MARALEE R. KANIN, MD
Endocrinology Fellow, Physician, Division of Endocrinology, Diabetes, and Metabolism, Department of Medicine, David Geffen School of Medicine, University of California, Los Angeles, Division of Endocrinology, Diabetes, and Metabolism, Department of Medicine, VA Greater Los Angeles Healthcare System, Los Angeles California, USA

AMANDA SILVER KARCIOGLU, MD
Division of Otolaryngology–Head and Neck Surgery, Department of Surgery, NorthShore University HealthSystem, Evanston, Illinois, USA

DIANA N. KIRKE, MD, MPhil, FRACS
Department of Otolaryngology–Head and Neck Surgery, Assistant Professor, Icahn School of Medicine at Mount Sinai, New York, New York, USA

PALLAVI KULKARNI, BS
Penn State Health Department of Otolaryngology–Head and Neck Surgery, Penn State College of Medicine, Hershey, Pennsylvania, USA

ANGELA M. LEUNG, MD, MSc
Associate Professor of Medicine, Division of Endocrinology, Diabetes, and Metabolism, Department of Medicine, David Geffen School of Medicine, University of California, Los Angeles, Associate Professor, Division of Endocrinology, Diabetes, and Metabolism, Department of Medicine, VA Greater Los Angeles Healthcare System, Los Angeles California, USA

KEVIN Y. LIANG, MD
Resident, Head and Neck Institute, Cleveland Clinic Foundation, Cleveland, Ohio, USA

LISA A. ORLOFF, MD
Professor, Department of Otolaryngology–Head and Neck Surgery, Stanford University, Stanford, California, USA

PIA PACE-ASCIAK, MASc, MD, FRCSC
Assistant Professor, Department of Otolaryngology–Head and Neck Surgery, Temerty Faculty of Medicine, University of Toronto, Toronto, Canada

GREGORY W. RANDOLPH, MD
Division of Thyroid and Parathyroid Endocrine Surgery, Department of Otolaryngology–Head and Neck Surgery, Massachusetts Eye and Ear Infirmary, Department of Surgery, Massachusetts General Hospital, Harvard Medical School, Boston, Massachusetts, USA

JONATHON O. RUSSELL, MD, FACS
Associate Professor, Director of Endoscopic and Robotic Thyroid and Parathyroid Surgery, Department of Otolaryngology–Head and Neck Surgery, Johns Hopkins School of Medicine, Baltimore, Maryland, USA

JOSEPH SCHARPF, MD
Professor, Head and Neck Institute, Cleveland Clinic Foundation, Cleveland, Ohio, USA

BRITNEY SCOTT, DO
Department of Surgery, Head and Neck Service, Memorial Sloan Kettering Cancer Center, New York, New York, USA

MAISIE SHINDO, MD
Professor, Department of Otolaryngology–Head and Neck Surgery, Director of Thyroid and Parathyroid Surgery, Director, Head and Neck Endocrine Surgery, Oregon Health and Science University, Portland, Oregon, USA

DAVID C. SHONKA Jr, MD
Division of Head and Neck Surgery, Department of Otolaryngology–Head and Neck Surgery, University of Virginia, Charlottesville, Virginia, USA

CATHERINE F. SINCLAIR, MD, FRACS, FACS
Department of Surgery, Monash University, Melbourne, Victoria, Australia; Department of Otolaryngology–Head and Neck Surgery, Icahn School of Medicine at Mount Sinai, New York, New York, USA; Associate Professor, Melbourne Thyroid Surgery, Malvern, Victoria, Australia

CRISTIAN M. SLOUGH, MD
Department of Otolaryngology–Head and Neck Surgery, Hawke's Bay Fallen Soldiers' Memorial Hospital, Te Whatu Ora Health New Zealand, Hastings, New Zealand

BRENDAN C. STACK Jr, MD, FACS, FACE
Former Inaugural Professor and Chairman, Department of Otolaryngology–Head and Neck Surgery, Southern Illinois University School of Medicine, Springfield, Illinois, USA

DAVID L. STEWARD, MD, FACS
Helen Bernice Broidy Professor and Chair, Department of Otolaryngology–Head and Neck Surgery, University of Cincinnati College of Medicine, Cincinnati, Ohio, USA

RAISA TIKHTMAN, MD
Resident Physician, Department of Otolaryngology–Head and Neck Surgery, University of Cincinnati College of Medicine, Cincinnati, Ohio, USA

NEIL TOLLEY, MD, FRCS, DLO
Department Otolaryngology–Head and Neck Surgery, St Mary's Hospital, Imperial College NHS Healthcare Trust, Paddington, London, United Kingdom

RALPH P. TUFANO, MD, MBA
Medical Director, Sarasota Memorial Health Care System Multidisciplinary Thyroid and Parathyroid Center, Sarasota, Florida, USA

RICHARD J. WONG, MD
Chief, Head and Neck Service, Department of Surgery, Memorial Sloan Kettering Cancer Center, New York, New York, USA

Contents

> The management of thyroid and parathyroid pathology varies widely, with unifying goals of symptomatic control and mitigating patient morbidity. In general, surgery is indicated when addressing malignancy or when medical management is insufficient. Over the last few decades, treatment paradigms for patients with head and neck endocrine disease have shifted significantly as our understanding of disease processes has expanded and with the advent of numerous relevant technologies. Here we provide a general overview of thyroid and parathyroid disease that may be managed by the otolaryngologist, with attention to emerging strategies in diagnosis and treatment.

> Thyroid and parathyroid disorders are quite common in the population and range from benign to malignant conditions that may be hormonally active or inactive. Select disorders of the thyroid and parathyroid can be managed medically, although there are a variety of circumstances that may require definitive management with surgery. Surgical intervention may be required for hormonal control, compressive symptoms, or for the removal and/or control of malignancy. The endocrinologist's perspective of the preoperative and postoperative management regarding thyroid and parathyroid surgeries will be discussed.

> Thyroidectomy is a surgical procedure to remove part or all of the thyroid gland. Although the general tenets of surgery have remained the same, improvements in techniques, diagnostics, understanding of anatomy, and technology have allowed thyroid surgery to become a standard, effective, and safe surgery. For surgeons undertaking this procedure, it is imperative to have an in-depth knowledge of critical anatomy and a comprehensive understanding of surgical techniques to perform safe and effective surgery. This article aims to provide an overview of surgical techniques that may be applied in both benign and malignant disease settings.

nodules has only emerged during the past 5 to 10 years in North America, RFA has an impressive track record of nodule reduction, compressive and cosmetic symptom improvement, and excellent safety profile without the morbidity of open surgery. The role of RFA in autonomous functioning nodules, thyroid cancer, and indeterminate nodules is controversial and remains an area of investigation.

Brendan C. Stack Jr.

Secondary hyperparathyroidism (SHPT) does not initiate as a primary dysfunction of parathyroid glands resulting from an intrinsic defect or disease but is the physiologic response of parathyroids to metabolic changes elsewhere in the body occurring over time. SHPT is a manifestation of a chronic condition that classically occurs from chronic kidney disease. In fact, given the relatively recent transition of populations from outside (agrarian) to indoor (industrial, information technology, and so forth) employment and a consequent reduction in sun exposure, combined with diets of highly processed food, vitamin D and calcium deficiencies are now the leading causes of SHPT.

Pallavi Kulkarni and David Goldenberg

Primary hyperparathyroidism is the most common cause of hypercalcemia, accounting for about 90% of all cases. This disorder is characterized by overactive parathyroid glands, leading to increased parathyroid hormone and excess serum calcium.

Catherine Alessandra Colaianni and Maisie Shindo

This guide delineates a step-by-step approach to targeted parathyroidectomy and 4 gland exploration, with embedded clinical pearls regarding anatomy, approach, and considerations.

Zoe H. Fullerton and Lisa A. Orloff

 Video content accompanies this article at http://www.oto.theclinics.com.

The treatment of hyperparathyroidism through parathyroidectomy requires careful and complete preoperative evaluation. There are multiple imaging modalities and methods available to clinicians today to aid in identifying a pathological lesion; however, each has limitations that the clinician must understand. A systematic approach to patient evaluation, imaging, and surgical exploration is necessary to ensure accurate diagnosis and maximize the chances of minimally invasive and successful surgical removal.

Postoperative hypoparathyroidism may cause significant patient morbidity and even mortality. Emerging technologies centered on autofluorescent properties of parathyroid glands when exposed to near-infrared light hold promise to improve surgical parathyroid gland identification and preservation. Two systems (probe-based and camera-based) are commercially available currently; however, neither system alone provides indication of vascular viability or postoperative parathyroid gland function. The administration of indocyanine green, when combined with near-infrared fluorescence imaging, enables subjective assessment of parathyroid gland perfusion. Additional technologies to assess parathyroid gland perfusion are being developed. The impact of these nascent technologies on relevant clinical outcomes is an area of active investigation.

The surgical management of thyroid and parathyroid disease has evolved considerably since the era of Theodor Kocher. We review the current trends in thyroid and parathyroid surgery concerning robotic surgery for remote access, the use of parathyroid autofluorescence detection technology to aid in the prevention of hypocalcemia as well as the use of thermal ablation to target thyroid nodules in a minimally invasive way. We also discuss how artificial intelligence is being used to improve the workflow and diagnostics preoperatively as well as for intraoperative decision-making. We also discuss potential areas where future research may enhance outcomes.

OTOLARYNGOLOGIC CLINICS
OF NORTH AMERICA

THE CLINICS ARE AVAILABLE ONLINE!
Access your subscription at:
www.theclinics.com

Foreword

When the Thyroid and Parathyroids Misbehave

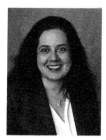

Sujana S. Chandrasekhar, MD, FAAO-HNS, FAOS, FACS
Consulting Editor

Thyroid surgery was first performed by the Moorish physician Abu Al Qasim Al Zahrawi, known in the West as Albucasis or Zahravius, in 952 AD. That procedure was recorded as the removal of a large goiter under sedation with opium with the use of simple ligatures along with hot cautery irons as the patient sat with a bag tied around his neck to collect the blood from the wound.[1] Unsurprisingly, the Roman encyclopedia reported that the operation to remove those masses in the anterior neck was simply too dangerous.

Interestingly and somewhat off-topic, Albucasis wrote a comprehensive textbook on medicine and surgery, which covered his innovations, including, among other areas, the following that pertain to Otolaryngology:

- A description of surgery of the eye, ear, and throat
- Full descriptions of tonsillectomy and tracheostomy
- A description of instruments he devised for the internal examination of the ear
- A description of an instrument he devised to be used to remove or insert objects into the throat
- A description of how to use a hook to remove a polyp from the nose
- A description of the exposure and division of the temporal artery to relieve certain types of headaches
- A description of the utilization of cauterization, usually to treat skin tumors or open abscesses, applying the cauterization procedure to as many as 50 different operations

Around 2700 BC, "goiter" was appreciated in China, and in as early as 1600 BC, the Chinese used burnt sponge and seaweed to treat goiters.[2] Pliny the Elder (AD23 to

Otolaryngol Clin N Am 57 (2024) xiii–xv
https://doi.org/10.1016/j.otc.2023.10.002
0030-6665/24/© 2023 Published by Elsevier Inc.

AD 79) noted goiter epidemics in the Alps and also mentioned the use of burnt seaweed in their treatment, which was supposedly learned from the Chinese. The *Atharva Veda* (2000 BC), an ancient Hindu collection of incantations, also contains exorcisms for goiter, which it called "galaganda." The Europeans began extirpation of the gland for suppuration or to apply dried or burnt seaweed in the eleventh century AD. It was not until 700 years later that it was determined that burning seaweed allows for a form of iodine treatment!

In 1511, Leonardo Da Vinci made the first anatomic drawing of the thyroid gland, but he was unsure of its function and thought it might just be a "spacer" between sternum and trachea. In the early seventeenth century, the thyroid gland was so named because of its appearance, which was similar to a shield, or *thyreos* in Greek. Even then, its function was not known, and it was thought to provide a rounded appearance to the neck in women.[3] Exophthalmic goiter was described by Parry of Bath in 1768, about 60 years before Graves and von Basedow separately published their findings.

Thyroidectomy outcomes were appalling for much of the eleventh to the nineteenth centuries. A thyroid surgeon who was the first to use a scalpel for this procedure, on a 10-year-old girl who subsequently died, was imprisoned in the mid-1600s for his work. Halsted identified a 40% mortality rate in thyroidectomies performed before 1850, and nearly all surgeons eschewed the procedure. The French Academy of Medicine enacted a complete ban on thyroidectomy in 1850. It was after that, with the advent of anesthesia, antisepsis, and hemostasis, that thyroidectomy began to emerge as a safe and effective procedure. Billroth saw his own mortality rate from this surgery reduce from 44% to 8.6% by 1881. His student, Kocher, further reduced that rate to 1% by 1895 and 0.5% by 1909, emphasizing extracapsular dissection. In 1909, Kocher won the Nobel Prize for his work on thyroid surgery.

And what of the parathyroid glands? They were first identified in a rhinoceros cadaver in 1852.[4] Their importance and methods to avoid damage to them or their blood supply were described in the early 1900s. Over time, parathyroid pathology independent of the thyroid was identified, and treatments were devised. Similarly, the effect of both goiter and surgery to address it on the voice was explored. The importance of the recurrent laryngeal nerves was obvious early on; it was not until a lead opera singer had an otherwise successful thyroidectomy in 1936 but subsequently lost her upper register and the ability to maintain the note, that the importance of the external branch of the superior laryngeal nerve was described. In the intervening nearly 90 years, we are still finding inadequate attention being paid to voice outcomes after thyroid and parathyroid surgery, leading to the publication of a Clinical Practice Guideline on behalf of the American Academy of Otolaryngology–Head and Neck Surgery on this topic.[5]

I went through this history because I believe this sets the stage for the current comprehensive issue of *Otolaryngologic Clinics of North America* on Thyroid and Parathyroid Disease, beautifully edited by Drs Amy Y. Chen and Michael C. Singer.

The articles they have included provide meaningful information, and the reader is sure to emerge from this issue able to offer even better care to their patients.

Sujana S. Chandrasekhar, MD, FAAO-HNS, FAOS, FACS
Consulting Editor, Otolaryngologic Clinics of North America
President, American Otological Society
Past President, American Academy of Otolaryngology-Head and Neck Surgery
Partner, ENT & Allergy Associates, LLP
Clinical Professor, Department of Otolaryngology-Head and Neck Surgery, Zucker
School of Medicine at Hofstra-Northwell
Clinical Associate Professor, Department of Otolaryngology-Head and Neck Surgery,
Icahn School of Medicine at Mount Sinai
18 East 48th Street, 2nd Floor
New York, NY 10017, USA

E-mail address:
ssc@nyotology.com

REFERENCES

1. Amr SS, Tbakhi A. Abu Al Qasim Al Zahrawi (Albucasis): pioneer of modern surgery. Ann Saudi Med 2007;27(3):220–1.
2. Sarkar S, Banerjee S, Sarkar R, et al. A review on the history of 'thyroid surgery. Indian J Surg 2016;78(1):32–6.
3. Ellis H. The early days of thyroidectomy. J Perioper Pract 2011;21(6):215–6.
4. Kalra S, Baruah MP, Sahay R, et al. The history of parathyroid endocrinology. Indian J Endocrinol Metab 2013;17(2):320–2.
5. Chandrasekhar SS, Randolph GW, Seidman MD, et al. Clinical practice guideline: improving voice outcomes after thyroid surgery. Otolaryngol–Head Neck Surg 2013;148:S1-37.

Preface

Thyroid and Parathyroid Surgery: No Longer "Horrid Butchery"

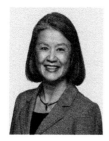 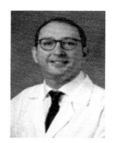

Amy Y. Chen, MD, MPH, MBA, FACS   Michael C. Singer, MD, FACS, FACE

Editors

Over the last several decades otolaryngologists have become increasingly involved in the care of patients with thyroid and parathyroid diseases. Endocrine surgery has become a key component of residency training, a significant element of many otolaryngologists' practices, and the sole focus of some practitioners. This same period has also seen a significant evolution in the practice of endocrine surgery—with advances in surgical procedures, adjunct technologies, and approaches to minimizing surgical risks. Modern thyroid and parathyroid surgery in many cases has become less invasive, safer, and more successful than traditional techniques.

In this issue of *Otolaryngologic Clinics of North America* these innovations are highlighted. Many of the articles focus on state-of-the-art approaches to traditional challenges, such as finding "missing" parathyroid glands or preserving the recurrent and superior laryngeal nerves. Other articles, like the one on parathyroid autofluorescence, discuss technologies and related techniques that potentially represent completely novel solutions to persistent surgical challenges.

Otolaryngol Clin N Am 57 (2024) xvii–xviii

https://doi.org/10.1016/j.otc.2023.08.003

0030-6665/24/© 2023 Published by Elsevier Inc.

oto.theclinics.com

We hope that regardless of the experience and knowledge of the reader this text will offer new ideas or concepts that will benefit surgeons and their future patients.

Amy Y. Chen, MD, MPH, MBA, FACS
Department of Otolaryngology Head and Neck Surgery
Emory University
550 Peachtree Street
Medical Office Tower, Suite 1135
Atlanta, GA 30308, USA

Michael C. Singer, MD, FACS, FACE
Division of Thyroid & Parathyroid Surgery
Department of Otolaryngology–
Head and Neck Surgery
Henry Ford Hospital
Detroit, MI 48202, USA

E-mail addresses:
achen@emory.edu (A.Y. Chen)
msinger@hfhs.org (M.C. Singer)

Overview of Thyroid and Parathyroid Disease
The Otolaryngology Perspective

Raisa Tikhtman, MD, David L. Steward, MD*

KEYWORDS

- Thyroid nodules • Thyroid cancer • Radiofrequency ablation • RFA
- Primary hyperparathyroidism • Minimally invasive

KEY POINTS

- The otolaryngologist may play a key role in the management of thyroid and parathyroid disease, requiring a nuanced understanding of multidisciplinary diagnostic and treatment approaches.
- Emerging strategies in the management of differentiated thyroid cancer emphasize de-escalation approaches to minimize patient morbidity without impairing oncologic outcomes.
- Minimally invasive approaches to thyroid and parathyroid surgery demonstrate rising popularity; however, care must be employed in patient selection.

INTRODUCTION

Within the vast realm of pathology that falls under the purview of Otolaryngology, the management of Head and Neck Endocrine disease is particularly nuanced and multidisciplinary. Thyroid surgery was pioneered in the late nineteenth century by Theodor Billroth and Theodor Kocher, with the latter ultimately receiving the Nobel Prize in Medicine and Physiology in 1909 to honor his achievements in illuminating thyroid pathology.[1] Initially the domain of general surgeons, otolaryngologists began performing thyroid and parathyroid surgery in the second half of the twentieth century. Endocrine surgery now comprises a foundational element of otolaryngologic surgical training and clinical practice.[2] Here, we provide an overview of surgical indications for benign and malignant thyroid and parathyroid disease as well as of emerging clinical practice trends for both domains.

Department of Otolaryngology–Head and Neck Surgery, University of Cincinnati College of Medicine, Medical Sciences Building Room #6507, 231 Albert Sabin Way, Cincinnati, OH 45267-0528, USA
* Corresponding author.
E-mail address: stewardd@ucmail.uc.edu

Otolaryngol Clin N Am 57 (2024) 1–9
https://doi.org/10.1016/j.otc.2023.07.003
0030-6665/24/© 2023 Elsevier Inc. All rights reserved.

BENIGN THYROID DISEASE

The otolaryngologist plays a role in the definitive management of a range of benign thyroid processes including hyperthyroidism secondary to toxic nodular disease or Graves' disease; hypothyroidism, either postoperative or acquired; and nodular thyroid disease.

Hyperthyroidism

The management of hyperthyroidism generally involves achieving symptomatic control and mitigating morbidity secondary to the underlying etiology. Graves' disease is the most common and often most severe cause of thyrotoxicosis, followed by toxic multinodular goiter and a single toxic adenoma.[3] Although patients may typically present to the otolaryngologist with a specific diagnosis for hyperthyroidism indicating a role for surgical management, the surgeon may in some cases be responsible for completing the diagnostic workup.

Clinical hyperthyroidism is defined by a low thyroid stimulating hormone (TSH;<0.4 mU/L) and an elevated free T_4 (FT_4) and/or T3 (free or total). If Graves' disease is suspected, serologic testing identifying the presence of TSH-receptor antibodies or thyroid-stimulating immunoglobulins confirms the diagnosis. Conversely, the presence of antibodies against thyroglobulin (Tg) or thyroid peroxidase is suggestive of Hashimoto's transient thyrotoxicosis. Thyroid uptake and scintigraphy can help to differentiate between conditions distinguished by TSH-receptor activation or autonomous thyroid hormone secretion versus destructive thyroiditis. In the setting of hyperfusion secondary to Graves' disease, toxic multinodular goiter, or a solitary toxic adenoma, the percentage of thyroidal uptake of the radiotracer will be increased. Conversely, in de Quervain thyroiditis, Hashimoto thyroiditis, and drug-induced conditions in which the thyrotoxicosis is self-limited, in the setting of an underlying inflammatory process inducing the release of preformed thyroid hormone, radiotracer uptake will be decreased on thyroid scintigraphy.[4] Patients who are pushed into thyrotoxicosis after receiving an exogenous iodine load, such as for contrasted computed tomography (CT) imaging, will likewise display low radioactive iodine uptake. Thyroid ultrasonography can also be helpful in distinguishing the underlying pathology for hyperthyroidism as well as identify existent or causative nodular disease. On ultrasonography, thyroid vascularity will be observed among patients with thyroid hyperfunction, whereas diminished vascularity is associated with destructive thyroiditis.[5]

Symptomatic hyperthyroidism is typically first addressed medically. Beta blockade can provide relief for patients with tachycardia, palpitations, or tremor. Antithyroid medications (methimazole or propylthiouracil) represent the first-line treatment of patients with Graves' disease, with the specific drug selection underlined by patient-specific factors. Although antithyroid therapy may be useful in the short term for patients with hyperthyroidism, they are not usually recommended long term due to myriad potential side effects. Furthermore, definitive therapy including radioactive iodine ablation (RAI) or surgery is often indicated to prevent disease progression.[4,6] RAI exhibits a cure rate of approximately 75% and is indicated in patients unable to tolerate antithyroid medications or who may not be candidates for surgery. RAI is also effective in the definitive treatment of toxic adenoma or toxic multinodular goiter, particularly when thyroid uptake is higher.[7]

Definitive surgical management may be indicated for patients with hyperthyroidism prefer it to antithyroid medications or have contraindications to their use. Graves' disease should be definitively managed with total thyroidectomy, which demonstrates a lower risk of recurrent hyperthyroidism than subtotal thyroidectomy; however, this approach necessitates a lifelong dependence on thyroid hormone supplementation. Toxic multinodular goiter with bilateral hyperfunctioning nodules may be similarly managed with total thyroidectomy. Patients with a single toxic adenoma are generally treated with hemithyroidectomy.

Radiofrequency ablation (RFA) represents a minimally invasive alternative for toxic adenomas which can mitigate some of the risks associated with RAI or surgery and may be indicated among patients who cannot tolerate either. RFA refers to the use of electrode needles directed under ultrasonographic guidance to induce coagulative necrosis of thyroid tissue. Fibrosis and nodule volume reduction ultimately arise within the treatment fields.[8] The procedure is typically performed on an outpatient basis using local anesthesia. Major complications are rare, affecting approximately 1% of patients.[9] Among patients with hyperfunctioning nodules, RFA may achieve up to 85% volume reduction and yield normalization of thyroid function tests in 24% to 86% of patients, with a greater benefit among those with smaller initial nodule size.[8,10]

Patients who elect to undergo surgery for hyperthyroidism must be optimized preoperatively to mitigate the risk of complications including thyroid storm. Furthermore, the surgeon must anticipate the greater intraoperative bleeding risk among Graves' patients due to the significantly increased vascularity of the thyroid gland. Patients should ideally achieve a euthyroid state (defined by normal or near-normal FT_4 and T3 testing) before surgery through several weeks of antithyroid medications. The American Thyroid Association's (ATA) guidelines recommend that most patients with Graves' disease also receive potassium iodide or Lugol's solution immediately preoperatively for the benefit of reducing thyroid vascularity and intraoperative blood loss. Five to seven drops of Lugol's solution may be mixed in water or juice and administered 3 times daily over the 7 to 10 days before surgery.[5]

Substernal Goiter and Thyroid Nodules

Substernal goiter describes an enlarged thyroid gland that extends inferior to the thoracic inlet, with more specific definitions varying widely within the literature.[11] Substernal goiters typically exhibit a slowly progressive course and are either discovered incidentally on imaging or present with compressive symptoms ranging from a mild cough to severe airway obstruction. They are usually associated with tracheal deviation and some degree of compression. In symptomatic patients with stridor and/or the inability to lay flat, an explicit airway plan before surgical intervention must be devised with the involvement of both the otolaryngologist and anesthesia team. Management is predominantly surgical, and the majority (>95%) may be approached transcervically, often with Thoracic Surgery on standby in case a sternotomy is required. Some surgeons may choose to stage hemithyroidectomies to mitigate the risk of injury to the bilateral recurrent laryngeal nerves depending on the extent of the disease.[12]

Thyroid nodules may be detected in up to 65% of the general population and are often identified incidentally on imaging obtained for other reasons. Although the vast majority of thyroid nodules are benign, 5% to 10% may harbor malignancy. About 95% of patients with thyroid nodules are asymptomatic, with the remaining 5% demonstrating compressive symptoms such as globus sensation, dysphagia, dysphonia, dyspnea, or pain.[13]

Management of thyroid nodules is dictated by sonographic features including size and other characteristics that may indicate the need for a biopsy via ultrasound-guided fine-needle aspiration (FNA). The ATA guidelines provide an algorithm for the evaluation and management of thyroid nodules based on sonographic findings and FNA cytology. In general, patients with benign (purely cystic) or low suspicion (spongiform or partially cystic without suspicious features) sonographic findings do not require FNA unless the nodule exceeds 2 cm.[14] Sonographically suspicious nodules necessitate biopsy at lower size thresholds, and the ATA guidelines recommend nodules with highly suspicious features to undergo diagnostic FNA when greater than or equal to 1 cm. Depending on institutional and individual practice patterns, the otolaryngologist may be responsible for performing thyroid ultrasounds and/or ultrasound-guided FNAs of thyroid lesions.

The Bethesda System outlines specific criteria for evaluating thyroid FNA cytopathology, with findings classified as benign (55%–75%), malignant (2%–5%), or cytologically indeterminate. Within the latter group, Bethesda findings may be reported as suspicious for malignancy (1%–6%), follicular neoplasm (2%–25%), and atypia of undetermined significance or follicular lesion of undetermined significance (2%–18%).[15] Patients with nodules of indeterminate cytology or Bethesda III or IV lesions may be offered diagnostic surgery or cytomolecular testing. Molecular testing typically involves a send-out test obtained from an FNA sample and may help to further stratify the risk of malignancy within the tested thyroid nodule. Mutational panels have expanded to include multiple genetic mutations and alterations beyond just *BRAF*, *NRAS*, *HRAS*, and *KRAS* and *RET/PTC1* and *RET/PTC3* translocations.[14] Molecular testing is useful to the otolaryngologist as a decision-making aid in the setting of indeterminate thyroid cytology. With a negative predictive value of approximately 95% among patients with Bethesda 3 and 4 cytology, molecular testing can help a significant number of patients avoid unnecessary diagnostic surgery.[16]

MALIGNANT THYROID DISEASE

The surgical management of thyroid malignancy is dictated by the histologic subtype and extent of the disease, with significant changes in treatment paradigms observed over the past few decades. Papillary thyroid carcinoma (PTC) is by far the most common thyroid malignancy and accounts for more than 80% of thyroid malignancy, followed by follicular thyroid carcinoma, Hurthle cell carcinoma, medullary thyroid cancer, and anaplastic thyroid carcinoma. Nearly half of the patients diagnosed with differentiated thyroid cancer will present with cervical lymph node involvement.[14,17] Thyroid and neck ultrasonography is an essential component of the preoperative evaluation, and the extent of cervical disease may be further delineated using CT imaging.

Historically, nearly all patients diagnosed with thyroid cancer underwent total thyroidectomy with or without neck dissection for malignant disease; however, current approaches have escalated therapy for low-risk cancer with an emphasis on minimizing patient morbidity. Accordingly, the ATA guidelines have outlined circumstances in which hemithyroidectomy may be appropriate for patients undergoing surgical treatment for low-risk thyroid cancer including unilobar PTC less than 4 cm without high-risk pathologic features.[14] The potential for needing a completion thyroidectomy as well as adjuvant RAI should be discussed with patients preoperatively.

Postoperatively, the otolaryngologist must use a modified risk stratification for patients who have undergone hemithyroidectomy rather than total thyroidectomy due to expected differences in Tg levels with an intact thyroid lobe. Following hemithyroidectomy, Tg is a less reliable metric for disease recurrence, and sonographic reevaluation becomes the mainstay of surveillance.[14]

Active surveillance represents another emerging strategy in the management of small, low-risk thyroid cancer. According to the 2015 ATA guidelines, active surveillance may primarily be offered to patients with low-risk tumors, namely papillary thyroid microcarcinomas (PTMC) (<1 cm) without evidence of local invasion or cervical metastases. Other patients that may be considered for this approach include those at high risk of perioperative complications, patients of advanced age, or those with a poor short-term prognosis secondary to severe comorbid conditions. These recommendations were supported by findings from 2 prospective studies from Japan demonstrating that 1465 patients with PTC followed via active surveillance for 15 years yielded similar disease-specific outcomes to patients who undergo surgical resection of PTMC.[18,19] A 2017 study by Kwon and colleagues reported retrospective findings of active surveillance among 192 patients with PTMC over a median 30 month follow-up. The authors noted overall low rates of tumor growth, with only 27 (14%) patients demonstrating a tumor size increase during follow up and 24 (13%) patients ultimately undergoing delayed thyroid surgery. Although there was no significant association between patient age and change in tumor size over the follow-up period, 4 patients displaying significant tumor growth were all less than 65 years old.[20] The growing body of evidence continues to support active surveillance as a viable strategy for appropriately selected patients in the management of low-risk PTC.[21]

RFA is a promising and increasingly popular alternative to surgery or active surveillance in the management of low-risk thyroid carcinoma. Zhang and colleagues[22] first demonstrated in 2016 that RFA was safe and effective at eliminating low-risk unifocal PTMC in a prospective study of 92 patients; however, the study was limited by a short (12 month) follow-up period. In a larger retrospective investigation of 133 patients with PTMC who underwent RFA and were followed for a mean of 39 months, no patients experienced recurrence or metastatic spread.[23] A recent systematic review and meta-analysis comparing outcomes of primary surgery versus RFA for low-risk PTMC demonstrated no difference in local, regional, or distant tumor recurrence between groups. A significantly higher complication rate was reported among patients receiving surgery versus RFA (7.8% and 3.3%, respectively; $p = 0.03$).[24] More recent studies have illustrated similar outcomes of RFA in the treatment of multifocal PTMC.[25,26] Although RFA remains a second-line option for the management of low-risk thyroid malignancy after surgery, it mitigates perioperative risk and offers the potential for disease eradication, unlike active surveillance.

PARATHYROID DISEASE

The otolaryngologist plays an integral role in the multidisciplinary management of parathyroid disease including sometimes in the initial workup of hypercalcemia. Primary hyperparathyroidism (PHPT) refers to the autonomous excess production of parathyroid hormone (PTH) by one or more parathyroid glands. PHPT is primarily a serologic diagnosis and requires laboratory evaluations to rule out other common etiologies for hypercalcemia. Patients with PHPT display high or inappropriately normal PTH levels, which should normally be suppressed in the setting of hypercalcemia. Obtaining 24 hour urine calcium helps to evaluate for familial hypocalciuric hypercalcemia (FHH), which involves a mutation in the renal calcium-sensing receptor and may present with chronic hypercalcemia. Distinct from patients with PHPT, patients with FHH display diminished urine calcium levels (<100 mg over 24 hours) as well as a calcium-to-creatinine clearance ratio less than 0.01. Important to note, normocalcemic PHPT represents a variant in which patients may display elevated PTH levels with normal total and ionized serum calcium in the absence of other serologic abnormalities or diagnostic concerns.[27] Patients should undergo comprehensive evaluations to rule out secondary etiologies for elevated PTH, including vitamin D deficiency, gastrointestinal malabsorption, chronic kidney disease (CKD), or renal calcium leak.

Historically, patients with suspected PHPT underwent bilateral neck exploration with the goal of identifying all 4 parathyroid glands to deduce which gland(s) appeared abnormal. As approximately 85% of patients with PHPT have a single adenoma, minimally invasive techniques that emphasize unilateral neck exploration when possible for the sake of minimizing patient morbidity surgical efficiency and augmenting surgical efficiency have become popularized.[28]

The first minimally invasive, endoscopic approach to parathyroidectomy was reported by Michel Gagner in 1996, after which there were numerous investigations into less invasive, video-assisted approaches to augment the efficiency of both thyroid and parathyroid surgery. With regards to parathyroid surgery, the advent of high-resolution ultrasonography, nuclear imaging (sestamibi scintigraphy and single photon emission computed tomography), and more recently 4 dimensional CT has allowed surgeons to more effectively identify the involved parathyroid quadrant preoperatively.[29] Minimally invasive approaches to parathyroidectomy may be curative in 97% to 99% of patients when intraoperative PTH testing is used.[27,30] A 50% reduction in the baseline PTH level 10 minutes after excision of the adenoma candidate is generally considered a successful result; however, a stricter criterion of an intraoperative PTH level of less than or equal to 40 pg/mL has been associated with the lowest persistent disease rates.[31] The parathyroid candidate may also be evaluated by the surgical pathologist intraoperatively to assess the degree of hypercellularity, weight of the excised gland, fat distribution, and for the presence of a normocellular parathyroid rim to aid in distinguishing between a normal parathyroid gland, hyperplasia, and adenoma.[32]

Although minimally invasive approaches to parathyroid adenoma excision are preferred, in some cases, bilateral neck exploration with the identification of all 4 parathyroid glands is necessary. Preoperative imaging studies may be nonlocalizing in 4.5% to 32% of cases, compromising the surgeon's ability to plan a focused cervical exploration.[33,34] Multiglandular parathyroid disease (double adenomas or hyperplasia) accounts for 15% to 20% of PHPT. Accordingly, insufficient reductions in intraoperative PTH levels after excision of a suspected parathyroid adenoma should indicate that additional glands may be involved.[35] Other indications for bilateral neck exploration with subtotal parathyroidectomy or total parathyroidectomy with parathyroid autotransplantation include PHPT among patients with multiple endocrine neoplasia 1, secondary hyperparathyroidism (typically due to CKD) refractory to medical management, and tertiary hyperparathyroidism.[36–38]

Over the past several decades, numerous strategies to aid in the intraoperative identification of parathyroid glands have been proposed with varying success. Preoperative intravenous methylene blue injection was first reported in 1971, with the benefits of being selectively absorbed by parathyroid tissue allowing for more rapid visualization of parathyroid glands.[39] Unfortunately, this strategy was marred by insufficient data to support widespread use and reports of neurotoxicity, particularly among patients taking serotonin reuptake inhibitors.[40] Intraoperative jugular venous sampling has demonstrated high (>75%) sensitivity for lateralizing the involved parathyroid gland but is generally reserved for cases with negative or discordant imaging or recurrent HPT.[41]

More recently, parathyroid autofluorescence, capitalizing on the unique autofluorescent ability of parathyroid tissue within the near-infrared (NIR) light spectrum, has become increasingly popular.[42] A fluorophore, typically indocyanine green (ICG), is injected intravenously and binds directly to plasma proteins within the intravascular space. With the aid of ICG as a contrast agent, the NIR autofluorescence of the parathyroid vasculature is more easily identified. Autofluorescence is detected intraoperatively using camera-linked probes which then translate findings within the surgical field to a screen, allowing the surgeon to compare their findings in real-time with those of the probe. Although parathyroid autofluorescence has demonstrated feasibility in numerous studies, its influence on clinical outcomes including recurrent laryngeal nerve injury and postoperative hypocalcemia remains unclear.[43]

SUMMARY

The otolaryngologist plays an integral role in the multidisciplinary management of thyroid and parathyroid disease, including diagnostically and surgically. Guidelines have been developed to help inform decision-making in the management of complex thyroid and parathyroid disease and should serve as a clinical reference and aid to the otolaryngologist. Current advancements in thyroid and parathyroid surgery emphasize surgical efficiency, improved patient disease control, and minimization of postoperative morbidity.

CLINICS CARE POINTS

- Hyperthyroidism is first treated medically, with ablative and surgical approaches reserved for patients unable to tolerate or contraindications to medical management.
- The management of thyroid nodules is dictated by size and associated compressive symptoms as well as cytopathology indicating risk of malignancy.
- Histologic subtype underlines surgical decision-making for patients with diagnosed thyroid malignancy, with a trend towards active surveillance among patients with small, low-risk disease.
- Minimally invasive surgical approaches to primary hyperparathyroidism are generally preferred, with numerous adjunctive strategies available to aid in disease localization.

DISCLOSURE

The authors have nothing to disclose.

REFERENCES

1. Sarkar S, Banerjee S, Sarkar R, et al. A review on the history of "thyroid surgery". Indian J Surg 2016;78(1):32–6.
2. Ramsden JD, Johnson AP, Cocks HC, et al. Who performs thyroid surgery: a review of current otolaryngological practice. Clin Otolaryngol Allied Sci 2002;27(5):304–9.
3. Goichot B, Caron P, Landron F, et al. Clinical presentation of hyperthyroidism in a large representative sample of outpatients in France: relationships with age, aetiology and hormonal parameters. Clin Endocrinol 2016;84(3):445–51.
4. Wiersinga WM, Poppe KG, Effraimidis G. Hyperthyroidism: aetiology, pathogenesis, diagnosis, management, complications, and prognosis. Lancet Diabetes Endocrinol 2023;11(4):282–98.
5. Ross DS, Burch HB, Cooper DS, et al. 2016 American thyroid association guidelines for diagnosis and management of hyperthyroidism and other causes of thyrotoxicosis. Thyroid 2016;26(10):1343–421.
6. van Soestbergen MJ, van der Vijver JC, Graafland AD. Recurrence of hyperthyroidism in multinodular goiter after long-term drug therapy: a comparison with Graves' disease. J Endocrinol Invest 1992;15(11):797–800.

7. Hughes K, Eastman C. Thyroid disease: Long-term management of hyperthyroidism and hypothyroidism. Aust J Gen Pract 2021;50(1–2):36–42.
8. Cesareo R, Palermo A, Pasqualini V, et al. Radiofrequency ablation on autonomously functioning thyroid nodules: a critical appraisal and review of the literature. Front Endocrinol 2020;11:317.
9. Kim C, Lee JH, Choi YJ, et al. Complications encountered in ultrasonography-guided radiofrequency ablation of benign thyroid nodules and recurrent thyroid cancers. Eur Radiol 2017;27(8):3128–37.
10. Sung JY, Baek JH, Jung SL, et al. Radiofrequency ablation for autonomously functioning thyroid nodules: a multicenter study. Thyroid 2015;25(1):112–7.
11. Wang LS. Surgical management of a substernal goiter. Formosan Journal of Surgery 2012;45(2):41–4.
12. Pieracci FM, Fahey TJ 3rd. Substernal thyroidectomy is associated with increased morbidity and mortality as compared with conventional cervical thyroidectomy. J Am Coll Surg 2007;205(1):1–7.
13. Durante C, Grani G, Lamartina L, et al. The diagnosis and management of thyroid nodules: a review. JAMA 2018;319(9):914–24.
14. Haugen BR, Alexander EK, Bible KC, et al. 2015 American thyroid association management guidelines for adult patients with thyroid nodules and differentiated thyroid cancer: the American thyroid association guidelines task force on thyroid nodules and differentiated thyroid cancer. Thyroid 2016;26(1):1–133.
15. Cibas ES, Ali SZ. The 2017 bethesda system for reporting thyroid cytopathology. Thyroid 2017;27(11):1341–6.
16. Alexander EK, Kennedy GC, Baloch ZW, et al. Preoperative diagnosis of benign thyroid nodules with indeterminate cytology. N Engl J Med 2012;367(8):705–15.
17. Nguyen QT, Lee EJ, Huang MG, et al. Diagnosis and treatment of patients with thyroid cancer. Am Health Drug Benefits 2015;8(1):30–40. Available at: https://www.ncbi.nlm.nih.gov/pubmed/25964831.
18. Sugitani I, Toda K, Yamada K, et al. Three distinctly different kinds of papillary thyroid microcarcinoma should be recognized: our treatment strategies and outcomes. World J Surg 2010;34(6):1222–31.
19. Ito Y, Miyauchi A, Kihara M, et al. Patient age is significantly related to the progression of papillary microcarcinoma of the thyroid under observation. Thyroid 2014;24(1):27–34.
20. Kwon H, Oh HS, Kim M, et al. Active surveillance for patients with papillary thyroid microcarcinoma: a single center's experience in Korea. J Clin Endocrinol Metab 2017;102(6):1917–25.
21. Smulever A, Pitoia F. Conservative management of low-risk papillary thyroid carcinoma: a review of the active surveillance experience. Thyroid Res 2023;16(1):6.
22. Zhang M, Luo Y, Zhang Y, et al. Efficacy and safety of ultrasound-guided radiofrequency ablation for treating low-risk papillary thyroid microcarcinoma: a prospective study. Thyroid 2016;26(11):1581–7.
23. Lim HK, Cho SJ, Baek JH, et al. US-guided radiofrequency ablation for low-risk papillary thyroid microcarcinoma: efficacy and safety in a large population. Korean J Radiol 2019;20(12):1653–61.
24. Kim HJ, Cho SJ, Baek JH. Comparison of thermal ablation and surgery for low-risk papillary thyroid microcarcinoma: a systematic review and meta-analysis. Korean J Radiol 2021;22(10):1730–41.
25. Yan L, Zhang M, Song Q, et al. Clinical outcomes of radiofrequency ablation for multifocal papillary thyroid microcarcinoma versus unifocal papillary thyroid

microcarcinoma: a propensity-matched cohort study. Eur Radiol 2022;32(2): 1216–26.

26. Teng DK, Li HQ, Sui GQ, et al. Preliminary report of microwave ablation for the primary papillary thyroid microcarcinoma: a large-cohort of 185 patients feasibility study. Endocrine 2019;64(1):109–17.

27. Wilhelm SM, Wang TS, Ruan DT, et al. The American association of endocrine surgeons guidelines for definitive management of primary hyperparathyroidism. JAMA Surg 2016;151(10):959–68.

28. Walsh NJ, Sullivan BT, Duke WS, et al. Routine bilateral neck exploration and four-gland dissection remains unnecessary in modern parathyroid surgery. Laryngoscope Investig Otolaryngol 2019;4(1):188–92.

29. Bunch PM, Kelly HR. Preoperative imaging techniques in primary hyperparathyroidism: a review. JAMA Otolaryngol Head Neck Surg 2018;144(10):929–37.

30. Milas M, Mensah A, Alghoul M, et al. The impact of office neck ultrasonography on reducing unnecessary thyroid surgery in patients undergoing parathyroidectomy. Thyroid 2005;15(9):1055–9.

31. Claflin J, Dhir A, Espinosa NM, et al. Intraoperative parathyroid hormone levels ≤40 pg/mL are associated with the lowest persistence rates after parathyroidectomy for primary hyperparathyroidism. Surgery 2019;166(1):50–4.

32. Cipriani NA, Glomski K, Sadow PM. Intraoperative assessment of parathyroid pathology in sporadic primary hyperparathyroidism: an institutional experience. Hum Pathol 2022;123:40–5.

33. Bergenfelz A, van Slycke S, Makay Ö, et al. European multicentre study on outcome of surgery for sporadic primary hyperparathyroidism. Br J Surg 2021; 108(6):675–83.

34. Chander NR, Chidambaram S, Van Den Heede K, et al. Correlation of preoperative imaging findings and parathyroidectomy outcomes support NICE 2019 guidance. J Clin Endocrinol Metab 2022;107(3):e1242–8. https://doi.org/10.1210/clinem/dgab740.

35. Kebebew E, Clark OH. Parathyroid adenoma, hyperplasia, and carcinoma: localization, technical details of primary neck exploration, and treatment of hypercalcemic crisis. Surg Oncol Clin N Am 1998;7(4):721–48. Available at: https://www.ncbi.nlm.nih.gov/pubmed/9735131.

36. Steinl GK, Kuo JH. Surgical management of secondary hyperparathyroidism. Kidney Int Rep 2021;6(2):254–64.

37. Palumbo VD, Palumbo VD, Damiano G, et al. Tertiary hyperparathyroidism: a review. Clin Ter 2021;172(3):241–6.

38. Schreinemakers JMJ, Pieterman CRC, Scholten A, et al. The optimal surgical treatment for primary hyperparathyroidism in MEN1 patients: a systematic review. World J Surg 2011;35(9):1993–2005.

39. Dudley NE. Methylene blue for rapid identification of the parathyroids. Br Med J 1971;3(5776):680–1.

40. Patel HP, Chadwick DR, Harrison BJ, et al. Systematic review of intravenous methylene blue in parathyroid surgery. Br J Surg 2012;99(10):1345–51.

41. Carneiro-Pla D. Contemporary and practical uses of intraoperative parathyroid hormone monitoring. Endocr Pract 2011;17(Suppl 1):44–53.

42. Paras C, Keller M, White L, et al. Near-infrared autofluorescence for the detection of parathyroid glands. J Biomed Opt 2011;16(6):067012.

43. Ladurner R, Lerchenberger M, Al Arabi N, et al. Parathyroid autofluorescence-how does it affect parathyroid and thyroid surgery? A 5 year experience. Molecules 2019;24(14). https://doi.org/10.3390/molecules24142560.

Overview of Thyroid and Parathyroid Disease—The Endocrinology Perspective

Maralee R. Kanin, MD[a,b], Angela M. Leung, MD, MSc[a,b],*

KEYWORDS

- Thyroid disease • Thyroid cancer • Thyroidectomy • Thyroid surgery
- Parathyroid disease • Primary hyperparathyroidism • Parathyroidectomy
- Parathyroid surgery

KEY POINTS

- Thyroid and parathyroid conditions can be benign or malignant, and hormonally active or inactive, for which medical management is often initially used.
- Thyroid and parathyroid diseases that may require surgical intervention include thyroid nodules (which may extend to obstructive or substernal goiter), hyperthyroidism, differentiated thyroid cancers (papillary, follicular, and oncocytic tumors of the thyroid), medullary thyroid cancers, anaplastic thyroid cancers, poorly differentiated and/or undifferentiated thyroid cancers, primary thyroid lymphomas, and metastatic disease from an extrathyroidal primary cancer.
- When medical treatment is prolonged, contraindicated, or financially prohibitive, alternative treatment is needed, including surgical resection.
- The management of thyroid and parathyroid diseases requires the coordination of a multidisciplinary team for optimal outcomes.

INTRODUCTION

Disorders of the thyroid and parathyroid include both benign and malignant conditions that may be hormonally active or inactive. When the duration of treatment is long, associated with high expense, required for the long-term, or not feasible, surgical resection is often the most effective means for definitive management of certain

a Division of Endocrinology, Diabetes, and Metabolism, Department of Medicine, David Geffen School of Medicine at University of California Los Angeles, 10833 Le Conte Avenue, CHS 57-145, Los Angeles, CA 90095, USA; b Division of Endocrinology, Diabetes, and Metabolism, Department of Medicine, VA Greater Los Angeles Healthcare System, 11301 Wilshire Boulevard (111D), Los Angeles CA 90073, USA
* Corresponding author. Division of Endocrinology, Diabetes, and Metabolism, Department of Medicine, VA Greater Los Angeles Healthcare System, 11301 Wilshire Boulevard (111D), Los Angeles, CA 90073.
E-mail address: amleung@mednet.ucla.edu

Otolaryngol Clin N Am 57 (2024) 11–24
https://doi.org/10.1016/j.otc.2023.07.007
oto.theclinics.com

thyroid and parathyroid disorders. The following is an endocrinologist's perspective for the preoperative and postoperative management of the select thyroid and parathyroid conditions that may require surgical intervention.

THYROID DISORDERS

Thyroid disorders range in scope and may include hormonally active conditions, benign or malignant tumors, and structural disorders. The conditions that may be indicated for surgical resection of the thyroid include thyroid nodules (which may extend to obstructive or substernal goiter), hyperthyroidism, differentiated thyroid cancers (papillary, follicular, and oncocytic tumors of the thyroid), medullary thyroid cancers (MTCs), anaplastic thyroid cancers, poorly differentiated and/or undifferentiated thyroid cancers, primary thyroid lymphomas, and metastatic disease from an extrathyroidal primary cancer. General indications for thyroid surgery include the need to alleviate compressive symptoms; tumor resection and/or to minimize the spread of metastatic thyroid cancer; and the need to achieve hormonal control for hyperthyroidism that is refractory to medical management. Proper workup with laboratory assessment and imaging, followed by medical management, is typically recommended before surgical intervention and will be discussed for each condition below (**Table 1**).

Hyperthyroidism

Thyrotoxicosis is the clinical syndrome that results when tissues are exposed to high levels of circulating thyroid hormones. The most common cause of hyperthyroidism worldwide is Graves disease, an autoimmune condition typically characterized by positive thyroid stimulating immunoglobulin (TSI) and/or thyrotropin receptor antibody (TRAb) titers that result in thyroid hormone overproduction. Other common causes of thyrotoxicosis include autonomously functioning thyroid nodule(s) and the thyrotoxic phase of thyroiditis, although both are less frequently encountered.

The diagnosis is typically confirmed with elevated serum levels of the peripheral thyroid hormones (thyroxine [T4] and/or triiodothyronine [T3]) and suppressed levels of thyroid stimulating hormone (TSH). Depending on the clinical suspicion of either Graves disease or one of the other causes of thyrotoxicosis, nuclear imaging with a thyroid uptake and scan (usually with the radioisotopes ^{123}I or technetium) may be needed, because a thyroid ultrasound may not demonstrate any thyroid nodules and serum thyroid antibodies that support Graves disease may or may not be positive. Graves disease is confirmed by diffusely increased uptake in the thyroid, whereas thyrotoxic thyroid nodules will display focally increased uptake, and the thyrotoxic phase of thyroiditis will show near absent uptake throughout the gland.

The medical treatment of Graves disease and autonomously functioning thyroid nodules is a thioamide (methimazole, carbimazole, or propylthiouracil) but may also include a beta-blocker for symptomatic relief in the initial 1 to 2 weeks. The duration of therapy is based on the etiology of the thyrotoxicosis and may extend up to 24 months for most cases of Graves disease but serve only as a temporizing measure for those with autonomously functioning thyroid nodules, for which definitive therapy is required.[1] Risks of thionamides include rash, hepatoxicity, and agranulocytosis.[2] For patients with Graves disease who require definitive treatment or patients with autonomously functioning thyroid nodules, radioactive iodine (RAI) therapy with orally administered ^{131}I is one consideration. Expected effects of RAI therapy include biochemical hypothyroidism, rather than restoration of euthyroidism. In patients with

Table 1
Diagnostic evaluation and management of conditions that may require thyroid surgery

Indication	Preoperative Evaluation	Preoperative Imaging	Indications for Thyroid Surgery	Postoperative Evaluation	Additional Considerations
Hyperthyroidism due to Graves disease	Serum TSH, T4, T3, TSI, and TRAb levels	Thyroid US; a thyroid radioactive uptake and scan may also be needed to confirm the diagnosis in select cases	≥2 y of antithyroid medication Contraindication to or side effect of antithyroid medication Plans for pregnancy in the next 6–12 mo Contraindication to RAI therapy	Postoperative serum TSH at 4–6 wk to adjust the LT4 dose as needed	
Hyperthyroidism due to autonomously functioning thyroid nodule(s)	Serum TSH, T4, and T3 levels	Thyroid US and RAI uptake and scan to localize the culprit nodule	Either a thyroid lobectomy, RAI therapy, or an ablative technique should be recommended for all confirmed autonomously functioning thyroid nodules	Postprocedural TSH at 4–6 wk to determine the need to start LT4	
Nonfunctional thyroid nodules and obstructive or substernal goiter	Serum TSH, FNA	Thyroid US and/or a neck/chest CT scan if unable to visualize the entire nodule	Either a thyroid lobectomy or total thyroidectomy is recommended if obstructive symptoms are present	Following partial thyroidectomy: Monitor TSH 4–6 wk postoperatively to determine the need to start LT4 Total thyroidectomy: Monitor TSH 4–6 wk postoperatively to adjust LT4 dose as needed	

(continued on next page)

Table 1
(continued)

Indication	Preoperative Evaluation	Preoperative Imaging	Indications for Thyroid Surgery	Postoperative Evaluation	Additional Considerations
Differentiated (papillary or follicular) cancer	Serum TSH, FNA	Thyroid US and/or CT scan if unable to visualize the nodule	Thyroid surgery (either as lobectomy or total thyroidectomy) should be generally recommended for all confirmed cases of differentiated thyroid cancer, except if the cancer is low-risk and the patient elects active surveillance of the malignancy	Following partial thyroidectomy: Monitor TSH 4–6 wk postoperatively to determine the need to start LT4. Total thyroidectomy: Monitor TSH 4–6 wk postoperatively to adjust LT4 dose as needed. Differentiated thyroid cancer surveillance with routine serum thyroglobulin and thyroglobulin antibody levels, and neck US	Genetic testing if there is evidence of a familial cancer syndrome (ie, familial adenomatous polyposis, Cowden syndrome, Carney complex, or familial papillary thyroid cancer)
MTC	Serum TSH, calcitonin, and CEA levels; FNA	Thyroid US	Total thyroidectomy	MTC surveillance with routine serum calcitonin and CEA levels, and neck US	Genetic testing and evaluation for MEN are recommended for all patients

Disease	Serum/biopsy tests	Imaging	Surgery	Postoperative management	Comanagement
Anaplastic thyroid cancer and poorly differentiated cancer	Serum TSH, FNA	Thyroid US Cross-sectional neck imaging is usually recommended to determine the extent of disease	Debulking thyroid surgery is usually needed to manage obstructive symptoms	Total thyroidectomy: Monitor TSH 4–6 wk postoperatively to adjust LT4 dose as needed	Comanagement with palliative care and oncology
PTL or metastatic disease from an extrathyroidal primary cancer	Serum TSH; thyroid peroxidase antibody is also recommended for PTL (though if inadequate, a core or surgical biopsy may be needed)	Thyroid US Cross-sectional imaging may be required to determine the extent of disease	Thyroid surgery is generally not the primary concern		Comanagement with oncology

Abbreviations: CEA, carcinoembryonic antigen; CT, computer tomography; FNA, fine needle aspiration; LT4, levothyroxine; MEN, multiple endocrine neoplasia; MTC, medullary thyroid cancer; PTL, primary thyroid lymphoma; RAI, radioactive iodine; T3, triiodothyronine; T4, thyroxine; TSH, thyroid stimulating hormone; US, ultrasound.

Graves disease who also have thyroid eye disease, RAI therapy may acutely worsen the eye disease and is thus usually contraindicated.[3]

Thyroidectomy is indicated for patients with disease refractory to thionamides and/or RAI therapy, severe liver impairment, preexisting agranulocytosis, and/or inability to tolerate thionamides; the desire to not receive RAI or have contraindications to RAI in some patients (ie, planned immediate pregnancy, thyroid eye disease); or a preference or need for surgical treatment to provide the most efficient resolution of thyrotoxicosis (ie, thyroid storm). In patients with Graves disease, a total thyroidectomy is preferred over subtotal thyroidectomy to reduce the risk of recurrence,[4] whereas a lobectomy is appropriate for those with autonomously functioning thyroid nodules. After a total thyroidectomy, full thyroid hormone replacement is needed and can be achieved with levothyroxine at a weight-based dosage of 1.6 mcg/kg/d. Monitoring of the serum TSH can be obtained at 4 to 6 weeks postoperatively to assess for the appropriateness of thyroid hormone replacement begun after a total thyroidectomy and for possible need to start thyroid hormone replacement after a thyroid lobectomy.

Nonfunctional Thyroid Nodules (Including Obstructive or Substernal Goiter)

Thyroid nodules are common and are increasingly prevalent with advancing age.[5] Thyroid nodules may be diagnosed on physical examination and often incidentally found on imaging for an alternative cause. The workup for a thyroid nodule includes obtaining a serum TSH to assess for possible hyperthyroidism and a dedicated thyroid ultrasound scan. Thyroid nodules are typically benign, with only less than 5% being malignant overall, although the risk of malignancy will vary by sonographic appearance.[6] Based on the sonographic risk assessment for malignancy, the decision to pursue possible fine needle aspiration (FNA) is made. Surgery may be recommended even for a benign thyroid nodule if there is a high risk of malignancy from the cytology result, or for those thyroid nodules that are large enough to cause compressive symptoms. Thyroid surgery would be recommended for malignant thyroid cytology, either as a lobectomy or total thyroidectomy.

Differentiated Thyroid Cancers

The prevalence of differentiated (papillary and/or follicular) thyroid cancers (DTCs) ranges from 5 to 17.6 per 100,000 patients.[7] Approximately 80% to 85% of thyroid cancers are papillary thyroid cancer. Middle-aged women tend to be affected in a 3 to 1 predominance compared with men.[8] Ionizing radiation exposure is one of the well-recognized risk factors for DTC, such as that incurred from frequent low-dose radiation in childhood or high-dose radiation associated with the treatment of malignancy, as well as a history of exposure to radiation fallout.

Thyroid nodules harboring cancer may be found incidentally during imaging for other indications or by physical examination. If a thyroid nodule is suspected, imaging with thyroid ultrasound should be obtained, in addition to consideration of aspiration of the nodule (with possible molecular testing if a cytologically indeterminate result is found) and measurement of serum TSH to rule out hyperthyroidism. Genetic testing is also advised for patients with family history of cancer syndromes such as familial adenomatous polyposis, Cowden syndrome, Carney complex, or familial papillary thyroid cancer.

Current guidelines advocate for a partial thyroidectomy for the initial treatment of low-risk DTCs. If, however, the pathologic condition demonstrates high-risk features such as extrathyroidal extension, angioinvasion or capsular invasion, or positive lymph nodes, completion thyroidectomy is usually performed.[6] In addition to a total thyroidectomy for intermediate-to high-risk cancers, RAI ablation may be recommended, and the dose of thyroid hormone replacement targeted to suppress the TSH to less than 0.1 mIU/L.[6] Long-term monitoring of DTC consists of serial serum thyroglobulin and thyroglobulin antibodies levels, in addition to surveillance neck ultrasounds.[6]

Medullary Thyroid Cancers

MTC is a much rarer type of thyroid cancer, accounting for around 4% of all thyroid cancers.[9] The defining feature of MTC is that it originates from the parafollicular cells of the thyroid and produces elevated serum calcitonin levels. Around 75% of MTC cases are sporadic, and the rest are associated with genetic conditions such as multiple endocrine neoplasia (MEN) types 2A and 2B.[10] Imaging, laboratory assessment for serum calcitonin levels, and FNA are required, and are obtained in the same process as described above for thyroid nodules suspected to harbor DTCs. In addition, genetic testing is advised in patients with first degree relatives of patients with hereditary MTC, parents whose children have classic phenotype of MEN2B, patients with cutaneous lichens amyloidosis, and adults with MEN2A and exon 10 mutations.[11] Total thyroidectomy is recommended for patients with high-risk genetic mutations.[12] Postoperatively, treatment should be started with thyroid hormone replacement to target a normal range serum TSH level. Serum calcitonin and carcinoembryonic antigen (CEA) levels should also be trended preoperatively and postoperatively to monitor for recurrence. Novel targeted therapies show promise for the treatment of recurrent and/or metastatic MTC.[13,14]

Anaplastic, Poorly Differentiated, and Undifferentiated Thyroid Cancers

Anaplastic thyroid carcinoma, also referred to as poorly differentiated or undifferentiated thyroid carcinoma, is another rare, highly aggressive malignant tumor. It accounts for approximately 2% to 3% of all thyroid gland neoplasms.[15] At time of diagnosis, there is usually already local invasion to the surrounding tissues, in up to 70% of patients.[15] The most common sites for local invasion include the trachea, esophagus, laryngeal nerve, and larynx. Lymph node metastases are seen in up to 40% of patients.[16] Metastatic disease can occur in up to 75% of patients, with the most common sites being the lungs, brain, and bones.[17]

The workup and management is similar to the above-mentioned thyroid cancers. In addition, PET scan also be obtained to evaluate overall disease burden. Prognosis is overall poor, and it is noted that most patients will pass from complications of obstruction or metastatic disease within in 1 year.[15] Surgical resection is still necessary to protect the airway and minimize the burden of disease, although it is not curative. Recent small studies suggest the potential benefit of targeted treatments and immunotherapies.[14] Palliative and oncologic consultations are also recommended.

Primary Thyroid Lymphomas and Metastatic Disease from Extrathyroidal Primary Cancers

Primary thyroid lymphoma (PTL) is quite rare and accounts for less than 5% of all thyroid cancers.[18] PTL refers to lymphoma that originates in the thyroid gland and then spreads to the lymph nodes. PTL can occur more commonly in patients with preexisting Hashimoto thyroiditis but there seems to be no association of PTL with other risk factors such as preexisting Graves disease, radiation exposure, preexisting nodules, or goiter.[19]

Patients typically present with a rapidly growing thyroid nodule and compressive symptoms. Serum thyroid function tests and antithyroid peroxidase antibodies can be obtained to evaluate for Hashimoto thyroiditis and possible hypothyroidism. If there is a high suspicion for PTL, imaging with computed tomography (CT) scan and/or MRI maybe more beneficial than a thyroid ultrasound to evaluate the extent of disease burden; a PET scan may also be obtained. FNA can be performed for evaluation by flow cytometry, although sampling may not be sufficient if there is only a small focus of lymphoma, and thus a core or an open surgical biopsy may be needed.[19] Treatment is with chemotherapy, which has been shown to rapidly reduce compressive symptoms; there is no role for surgical resection in this condition.[19]

PARATHYROID DISEASE

Parathyroid disorders are typically less common than thyroid disorders. Parathyroid surgeries are typically required for malignancy and hyperparathyroidism. Specifically, the conditions that may require surgical intervention include primary hyperparathyroidism (PHPT), secondary hyperparathyroidism, tertiary hyperparathyroidism, parathyroid carcinomas, and parathyroid cysts (**Table 2**).

Primary Hyperparathyroidism

PHPT affects approximately 1 to 7 cases per 1000 adults.[20] It is 2 to 3 times more common in women and the elderly population, compared with men.[20] PHPT originates from autonomous overproduction of parathyroid hormone (PTH) by one or more abnormal parathyroid glands, which may result in hypercalcemia, although normocalcemic PHPT is also possible.[21] This latter entity is thought to be a milder form of autonomous parathyroid function because the laboratory evaluation reveals concurrently normal calcium and elevated PTH levels. Symptoms from PHPT are from the hypercalcemia, which include polydipsia and polyuria, nephrolithiasis or nephrocalcinosis, pancreatitis, peptic ulcer disease or gastroesophageal reflux, neurocognitive dysfunction, or neuropsychiatric symptoms.

The diagnosis of PHPT is confirmed with laboratory assessment.[22] The biochemical criterion for classic PHPT requires a total serum calcium of more than 1.0 mg/dL (0.25 mmol/L) greater than the upper limit of normal and an elevated or inappropriately normal (ie, nonsuppressed) PTH level. Further evaluation should include the assessment of hypercalciuria (24-hour urine calcium level >400 mg/dL) and impaired renal function (glomerular filtration rate [GFR] <60 mL/min) to determine end-organ involvement. Similarly, imaging evaluation for end-organ involvement includes all of the following: Dual energy x-ray absorptiometry (DXA) to evaluate for osteoporosis (defined as a T-score of <−2.5), X-ray of the spine to evaluate for vertebral compression fractures, and renal ultrasound to evaluate for kidney stones. To localize the disease, neck ultrasonography, parathyroid sestamibi scan, and/or 4-dimensional CT can be used.[23]

Parathyroidectomy of the candidate parathyroid adenoma is indicated for all patients with PHPT who have any evidence of end-organ involvement, as ascertained from the above testing. Postoperatively, it is necessary to monitor serum calcium levels because transient hypocalcemia may occur due to hungry bone syndrome. Genetic testing is indicated in those who are at high-risk for mutations, such as those with familial hyperparathyroidism, family history of other personal comorbidities concerning for MEN 1 or 2 syndrome, or a family history of parathyroid cancer. Approximately 85% of PHPT is sporadic.[24]

Secondary Hyperparathyroidism

Secondary hyperparathyroidism can develop in patients with chronic kidney disease because of underlying and persistent hypocalcemia, hyperphosphatemia, and vitamin

Table 2
Diagnostic evaluation and management of conditions that may require parathyroid surgery

Indication	Preoperative Evaluation	Preoperative Imaging	Indications for Parathyroid Surgery	Postoperative Evaluation	Additional Considerations
PHPT	Serum calcium, albumin, PTH, 25OHD, BMP, 24-h urine calcium and creatinine	Localizing imaging with a sestamibi parathyroid scan, neck US, or 4D CT Other imaging to determine end-organ involvement: Spinal X-ray, DXA, renal US	Biochemical abnormalities: Serum calcium > 1.0 mg/dL (0.25 mmol/L) above the upper limit of the reference range; hypercalciuria (24-h urine calcium >400 mg/dL); impaired renal function (GFR <60 mL/min) Imaging abnormalities: DXA showing osteoporosis (T-score <−2.5) at the spine, hip, and/or forearm; evidence of fracture Nephrolithiasis observed either clinically or by renal US Surgery is indicated if there are symptoms referable to hypercalcemia	Serum calcium and PTH in the immediate postoperative period, then annually thereafter	Genetic testing for MEN if there is personal or family history of familial hyperparathyroidism or relevant components of the syndrome
Secondary hyperparathyroidism	Serum calcium, albumin, PTH, phosphorus, 25OHD, and creatinine	Relevant imaging to rule out a dominant parathyroid adenoma (sestamibi parathyroid scan, neck US, or 4D CT)	PTH >800 pg/mL for >6 mo despite medical intervention Persistent hypercalcemia: corrected serum calcium >10.2 mg/dL [>2.5 mmol/L] Persistent hyperphosphatemia: phosphorus >5.5 mg/dL [>1.8 mmol/L] Elevated risk or presence of calciphylaxis	Serial monitoring of the same panel as the preoperative laboratory parameters	

(continued on next page)

Table 2
(continued)

Indication	Preoperative Evaluation	Preoperative Imaging	Indications for Parathyroid Surgery	Postoperative Evaluation	Additional Considerations
Tertiary hyperparathyroidism	Serum calcium, albumin, PTH, phosphorus, 25OHD and creatinine	Relevant imaging to rule out a dominant parathyroid adenoma (sestamibi parathyroid scan, neck US, or 4D CT)	Persistent hypercalcemia and elevated PTH levels >1 y despite aggressive medical management with active vitamin D, phosphate binders, and calcimimetics	Serial serum calcium levels, targeting normal levels at 6 mo postoperatively	
Parathyroid carcinoma	Serum calcium, albumin, PTH, phosphorus, and 25OHD	Neck US and/or 4D CT	Surgical resection is usually performed for a suspicious structure and/or severe hypercalcemia, and the diagnosis is confirmed pathologically	Serial serum calcium, albumin, and PTH	Genetic testing if there is a family history of parathyroid carcinoma
Parathyroid cyst	Serum calcium, albumin, PTH, phosphorus and 25OHD	Neck US to consider the need for US-guided drainage	Surgical resection is usually performed for functional cysts, recurrent cysts, or if obstructive symptoms are present	Monitor for recurrence with serial US scans	

Abbreviations: 25OHD, 25-hydroxy vitamin D; BMP, basic metabolic panel; Cr, creatinine; CT, computed tomography; DXA, dual-energy X-ray absorptiometry; MEN, multiple endocrine neoplasia; PTH, parathyroid hormone; US, ultrasound.

D deficiency. This condition is present in nearly all patients at the time of initiation of dialysis. Typically, these patients are managed medically with active vitamin D and calcimimetics. Serum PTH levels in dialysis patients are typically kept within the range of 60 to 240 ng/mL, although there is no consensus of an optimal PTH level at which bone disease may be prevented.[25]

Parathyroidectomy is indicated in patients with refractory secondary hyperparathyroidism, such as that associated with hypercalcemia, hyperphosphatemia, or severe symptoms of hypercalcemia, despite aggressive medical intervention.[26] Aggressive medical intervention includes active vitamin D, phosphate binders, and calcimimetics. Laboratory criteria that are generally accepted for parathyroidectomy in such patients include a PTH greater than 800 pg/mL for more than 6 months despite medical intervention, persistent hypercalcemia (ie, corrected serum calcium >10.2 mg/dL [>2.5 mmol/L]), hyperphosphatemia (ie, phosphorus >5.5 mg/dL [>1.8 mmol/L]), elevated risk or presence of calciphylaxis, and erythropoietin-resistant anemia when other modifiable factors have been ruled out.[26] Preoperative imaging with four-dimensional (4D) CT scanning is often recommended.

Tertiary Hyperparathyroidism

Tertiary hyperparathyroidism develops in patients with preexisting secondary hyperparathyroidism or is defined as hyperparathyroidism that persists for more than 1 year after successful renal transplantation. Diagnosis is confirmed by elevated serum calcium and PTH levels in such patients. Prolonged PTH elevations in renal transplant recipients is associated with an increased risk of allograft failure, bone loss, increased vascular calcification, increased risk of cardiovascular events, and decreased patient survival.[27]

Historically, tertiary hyperparathyroidism has been treated with surgery with either subtotal or total parathyroidectomy, with or without autotransplantation.[27] Cinacalcet, although not approved by the US Federal Drug Administration for the treatment of tertiary hyperparathyroidism, is used off-label as the first-line medical management. Cinacalcet has been shown to be effective in the short term; however, long-term data are lacking, and cost may be prohibitive.[28] Before surgical intervention, there must be a trial of aggressive medical management with active vitamin D, phosphate binders, and calcimimetics.[27] If there is persistent, symptomatic hypercalcemia despite these therapies, surgery is needed for definitive treatment, although there is no specific PTH threshold with which parathyroid surgery is recommended.[25] Preoperative imaging is typically performed but it has been observed that preoperative imaging in tertiary hyperparathyroidism may not accurately localize all the abnormal parathyroid glands or ectopic glands.[29] The goal of surgery is to achieve a normal serum calcium level at 6 months postoperatively.

Parathyroid Carcinomas

Parathyroid carcinoma is a rare malignancy. The prevalence is around 0.005% of all malignancies and the annual incidence is ~3.5 to 5.7 cases per 10,000,000 population.[30] Parathyroid carcinoma is classified as localized, metastatic, or recurrent and defined pathologically by the presence of invasion into surrounding structures and/or the presence of distant disease.[31] Typically, clinical presentation develops from symptomatic hypercalcemia. Although there are no specific tumor markers for parathyroid carcinoma, preoperative biochemical testing should include serum calcium, PTH, phosphorus, albumin, and vitamin D levels. Serum calcium levels are often severely elevated (ie, >14 mg/dL), and PTH levels are typically at least 3 times greater than the upper limit of the normal range. Imaging with 4D CT is recommended preoperatively, and genetic screening can be performed if there is a family history of parathyroid cancer.

Parathyroid Cysts

Parathyroid cysts are exceedingly rare comprising less than 1% of neck masses and 0.5% to 1% of all parathyroid lesions.[32] Parathyroid cysts are classified as either functional or nonfunctional for the secretion of PTH, and some cysts may also harbor a parathyroid carcinoma. Diagnostic workup includes the biochemical evaluation for serum PTH, calcium, albumin, phosphorus, and vitamin D levels. FNA is the first step in management because this can be both diagnostic and curative.[33] Surgical resection is reserved for functional parathyroid cysts, recurrent parathyroid cysts, or if obstructive symptoms are present.[34]

SUMMARY

Thyroid and parathyroid disorders range from benign to malignant conditions to hormonally active. When medical treatment is not feasible, cost prohibitive, or there is structural compromise, surgical management is often the preferred means for definitive management.

CLINICS CARE POINTS

- Conditions of the thyroid that may require surgical resection include thyroid nodules/ obstructive or substernal goiter, hyperthyroidism, differentiated (papillary or follicular) thyroid cancer, MTC, anaplastic thyroid cancer, poorly differentiated and/or undifferentiated thyroid cancers, and PTL, metastatic disease of the thyroid from extrathyroidal primary cancer.
- The general indications for thyroid surgery include the alleviation of compressive symptoms, tumor resection and/or to minimize spread of metastatic cancer, and to achieve hormonal control in hyperthyroidism that is refractory or not amenable to medical management.
- The parathyroid conditions that may require surgical intervention include PHPT, secondary hyperparathyroidism, tertiary hyperparathyroidism, parathyroid carcinomas, and parathyroid cysts.

CONFLICT OF INTEREST STATEMENT

The authors have no commercial or financial interests to disclose.

REFERENCES

1. Ross DS, Burch HB, Cooper DS, et al. 2016 American Thyroid Association Guidelines for Diagnosis and Management of Hyperthyroidism and Other Causes of Thyrotoxicosis. Thyroid 2016;26(10):1343–421.
2. Bandyopadhyay U, Biswas K, Banerjee RK. Extrathyroidal actions of antithyroid thionamides. Toxicol Lett 2002;128(1–3):117–27.
3. Ariamanesh S, Ayati N, Mazloum Khorasani Z, et al. Effect of Different 131I Dose Strategies for Treatment of Hyperthyroidism on Graves' Ophthalmopathy. Clin Nucl Med 2020;45(7):514–8.
4. Guo Z, Yu P, Liu Z, et al. Total thyroidectomy vs bilateral subtotal thyroidectomy in patients with Graves' diseases: a meta-analysis of randomized clinical trials. Clin Endocrinol 2013. https://doi.org/10.1111/cen.12209.

5. Mazzaferri EL. Management of a solitary thyroid nodule. N Engl J Med 1993; 328(8):553–9.
6. Haugen BR, Alexander EK, Bible KC, et al. 2015 American Thyroid Association Management Guidelines for Adult Patients with Thyroid Nodules and Differentiated Thyroid Cancer: The American Thyroid Association Guidelines Task Force on Thyroid Nodules and Differentiated Thyroid Cancer. Thyroid 2016;26(1):1–133.
7. Kitahara CM, Sosa JA, Shiels MS. Influence of Nomenclature Changes on Trends in Papillary Thyroid Cancer Incidence in the United States, 2000 to 2017. J Clin Endocrinol Metab 2020;105(12):e4823–30.
8. Aschebrook-Kilfoy B, Grogan RH, Ward MH, et al. Follicular thyroid cancer incidence patterns in the United States, 1980-2009. Thyroid 2013;23(8):1015–21.
9. Hirsch D, Twito O, Levy S, et al. Temporal Trends in the Presentation, Treatment, and Outcome of Medullary Thyroid Carcinoma: An Israeli Multicenter Study. Thyroid 2018;28(3):369–76.
10. Cosway B, Fussey J, Kim D, et al. Sporadic medullary thyroid cancer: a systematic review and meta-analysis of clinico-pathological and mutational characteristics predicting recurrence. Thyroid Res 2022;15(1):12.
11. Wells SA, Asa SL, Dralle H, et al. Revised American Thyroid Association guidelines for the management of medullary thyroid carcinoma. Thyroid 2015;25(6): 567–610.
12. Elisei R, Romei C, Renzini G, et al. The timing of total thyroidectomy in RET gene mutation carriers could be personalized and safely planned on the basis of serum calcitonin: 18 years experience at one single center. J Clin Endocrinol Metab 2012;97(2):426–35.
13. Opsahl EM, Akslen LA, Schlichting E, et al. Trends in Diagnostics, Surgical Treatment, and Prognostic Factors for Outcomes in Medullary Thyroid Carcinoma in Norway: A Nationwide Population-Based Study. Eur Thyroid J 2019;8(1):31–40.
14. Al-Jundi M, Thakur S, Gubbi S, et al. Novel Targeted Therapies for Metastatic Thyroid Cancer-A Comprehensive Review. Cancers 2020;12(8):2104.
15. Nagaiah G, Hossain A, Mooney CJ, et al. Anaplastic thyroid cancer: a review of epidemiology, pathogenesis, and treatment. J Oncol 2011;2011:542358.
16. Giuffrida D, Gharib H. Anaplastic thyroid carcinoma: Current diagnosis and treatment. Ann Oncol 2000;11(9):1083–90.
17. Polistena A, Monacelli M, Lucchini R, et al. The role of surgery in the treatment of thyroid anaplastic carcinoma in the elderly. Int J Surg Lond Engl 2014;12(Suppl 2):S170–6.
18. Lee JS, Shin SJ, Yun HJ, et al. Primary thyroid lymphoma: A single-center experience. Front Endocrinol 2023;14:1064050.
19. Walsh S, Lowery AJ, Evoy D, et al. Thyroid lymphoma: recent advances in diagnosis and optimal management strategies. Oncol 2013;18(9):994–1003.
20. Yeh MW, Ituarte PHG, Zhou HC, et al. Incidence and prevalence of primary hyperparathyroidism in a racially mixed population. J Clin Endocrinol Metab 2013; 98(3):1122–9.
21. Cusano NE, Cetani F. Normocalcemic primary hyperparathyroidism. Arch Endocrinol Metab 2022;66(5):666–77.
22. Wilhelm SM, Wang TS, Ruan DT, et al. The American Association of Endocrine Surgeons Guidelines for Definitive Management of Primary Hyperparathyroidism. JAMA Surg 2016;151(10):959–68.
23. Bilezikian JP, Khan AA, Potts JT. Guidelines for the Management of Asymptomatic Primary Hyperparathyroidism: Summary Statement from the Third International Workshop. J Clin Endocrinol Metab 2009;94(2):335–9.

24. Park HS, Lee YH, Hong N, et al. Germline Mutations Related to Primary Hyper-parathyroidism Identified by Next-Generation Sequencing. Front Endocrinol 2022;13:853171.

25. Kidney Disease. Improving Global Outcomes (KDIGO) CKD-MBD Update Work Group. KDIGO 2017 Clinical Practice Guideline Update for the Diagnosis, Evaluation, Prevention, and Treatment of Chronic Kidney Disease-Mineral and Bone Disorder (CKD-MBD). Kidney Int Suppl 2017;7(1):1–59.

26. Lau WL, Obi Y, Kalantar-Zadeh K. Parathyroidectomy in the Management of Secondary Hyperparathyroidism. Clin J Am Soc Nephrol CJASN 2018;13(6):952–61.

27. Dulfer RR, Franssen GJH, Hesselink DA, et al. Systematic review of surgical and medical treatment for tertiary hyperparathyroidism. Br J Surg 2017;104(7):804–13.

28. Dulfer RR, Koh EY, van der Plas WY, et al. Parathyroidectomy versus cinacalcet for tertiary hyperparathyroidism; a retrospective analysis. Langenbeck's Arch Surg 2019;404(1):71–9.

29. Wang R, Abraham P, Lindeman B, et al. Is preoperative parathyroid localization necessary for tertiary hyperparathyroidism? Am J Surg 2022;224(3):918–22.

30. Ullah A, Khan J, Waheed A, et al. Parathyroid Carcinoma: Incidence, Survival Analysis, and Management: A Study from the SEER Database and Insights into Future Therapeutic Perspectives. Cancers 2022;14(6):1426.

31. Fingeret AL. Contemporary Evaluation and Management of Parathyroid Carcinoma. JCO Oncol Pract 2021;17(1):17–21.

32. Ippolito G, Palazzo FF, Sebag F, et al. A single-institution 25-year review of true parathyroid cysts. Langenbeck's Arch Surg 2006;391(1):13–8.

33. Ruiz J, Ríos A, Rodríguez JM, et al. Non-Functioning Parathyroid Cysts Refractory to Conservative Treatment. Cir Esp Engl Ed 2018;96(1):52–4.

34. Román-González A, Aristizábal N, Aguilar C, et al. Parathyroid cysts: the Latin-American experience. Gland Surg 2016;5(6):559–64.

Step-by-Step Thyroidectomy—Incision, Nerve Identification, Parathyroid Preservation, and Gland Removal

Britney Scott, DO, Richard J. Wong, MD*

KEYWORDS

- Hemithyroidectomy • Lobectomy • Thyroidectomy • Recurrent laryngeal nerve
- Parathyroid

KEY POINTS

- Surgery plays a central role for a variety of pathologic conditions of the thyroid gland including benign, malignant, and hormonal disease processes.
- Knowledge of surgical anatomy is essential to perform a safe and effective surgery with the goal of avoiding postsurgical complications such as vocal cord paralysis, postoperative hypocalcemia, or hematoma.
- Special attention to key anatomic areas during surgery will help the surgeon to avoid leaving residual thyroid tissue behind. These areas include the pyramidal lobe, upper pole, and Berry ligament.

INTRODUCTION

Thyroidectomy is a surgical procedure to remove part or all of the thyroid gland. Surgical techniques have advanced since the procedure was originally described in 1870. Although the general tenets of surgery have remained the same, improvements in techniques, diagnostics, understanding of anatomy, and technology have allowed thyroid surgery to become a standard, effective, and safe surgery.[1]

For surgeons undertaking this procedure, it is imperative to have an in-depth knowledge of critical anatomy and a comprehensive understanding of surgical techniques to perform safe and effective surgery. Although there are multiple different surgical techniques to perform this procedure, this article aims to provide an overview of surgical techniques that may be applied in both benign and malignant disease settings.

Head and Neck Service, Department of Surgery, Memorial Sloan Kettering Cancer Center, New York, NY 10021, USA
* Corresponding author. Memorial Sloan Kettering Cancer Center, New York, NY 10021.
E-mail address: wongr@mskcc.org

Otolaryngol Clin N Am 57 (2024) 25–37
https://doi.org/10.1016/j.otc.2023.08.007
0030-6665/24/© 2023 Elsevier Inc. All rights reserved.

SURGICAL INDICATIONS

Surgery plays a central role for a variety of pathologic conditions of the thyroid gland including benign, malignant, and hormonal disease processes. A complete review of the general indications for surgery is beyond the scope of this article but can be reviewed in the most recent edition of the American Thyroid Association guidelines and in other articles of this issue.[2] Decisions on indications for surgery and the extent of thyroidectomy can vary between surgeon and patient preferences, as well as institutional practices. In general, a discussion between the surgeon, endocrinologist, and patient is imperative to determine the best course of action. Factors influencing the extent of surgery are best made based on the initial extent of disease, prognostic factors, risk group stratification, and anticipated need for radioactive iodine (RAI) in the setting of differentiated thyroid carcinoma.[2–6]

GOALS OF SURGERY

The goal of surgery in the treatment of thyroid pathologic conditions is aimed at performing a thorough and safe operation with the least potential influence on the patient's quality of life. Special attention to preservation of the recurrent laryngeal nerve (RLN) and its branches, parathyroid glands, and removal of all gross thyroid tissue is needed to achieve these goals. The last point is particularly important in the setting of treatment of thyroid carcinoma or for tumors suspected to be cancerous. In this setting, the aim of surgical resection should be to achieve gross total clearance of all demonstrable disease (R0 resection). This is achieved through performing a total extracapsular dissection without leaving any residual thyroid tissue in the surgical bed paying special attention to the pyramidal lobe, the upper pole, and the region of Berry ligament.[7,8]

STEP-BY-STEP THYROIDECTOMY AND SURGICAL ANATOMY PEARLS ALONG THE WAY
Incision

The ideal incision should nearly always be planned in a natural skin crease (**Fig. 1**). A wider incision within a natural skin crease is cosmetically preferred over a smaller incision at a site lacking a crease. A smaller incision is generally more feasible if the

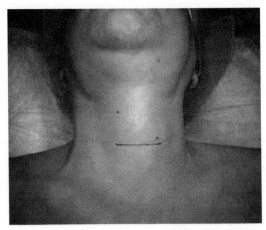

Fig. 1. The incision is placed in a natural skin crease approximately 4 cm in length.

incision is placed near the cricoid cartilage, although the shape and size of the thyroid gland influences the incision location. The length of the incision depends on multiple factors including the size of the thyroid, the size of the thyroid lesion, the patient's neck anatomy, and the need to remove lymph nodes.

Flap Elevation

The incision is carried down through the skin, subcutaneous fat, and platysma muscle, which is absent in the midline. Once the platysma is transected, superior and inferior subplatysmal flaps are elevated in the plane of the investing fascia, which is avascular (**Fig. 2**). Subcutaneous fat is typically elevated on the undersurface of the platysma, which is lifted, whereas the fascia is maintained intact over the anterior jugular veins and sternohyoid muscles. The flap is elevated superiorly to the middle portion of the thyroid cartilage and inferiorly carried down to the level of the lower pole of the thyroid gland. Care should be taken to avoid inadvertent injury to the anterior jugular veins. Some surgeons may elect to not elevate a subplatysmal flap and proceed directly to dividing the midline fascia.

Thyroid Gland Exposure

The subplatysmal skin flaps can be retracted using yellow hooks, which are positioned in the subcutaneous tissues to protect the skin edges. The surgeon will then encounter the underlying strap musculature—sternohyoid superficially followed by the sternothyroid. The fascia over the strap muscles is incised in the midline (**Fig. 3**), and the sternohyoid muscle is retracted laterally to expose the underlying sternothyroid muscle and anterior capsule of the thyroid gland (**Fig. 4**). Care should be taken when dissecting the muscles to grasp just the overlying fascia of the muscles to avoid unnecessary injury and bleeding from the muscle fibers. If the surgeon is performing a thyroidectomy to remove a potential cancer, the thyroid gland should be lightly palpated to identify the location of the tumor and to ensure there is no extracapsular extension

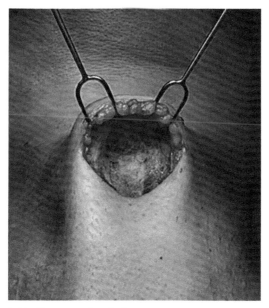

Fig. 2. Subplatysmal skin flaps are elevated.

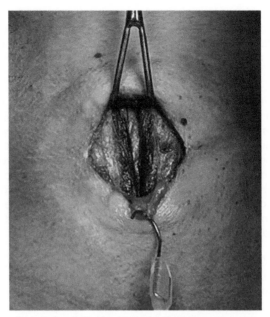

Fig. 3. The midline raphe is divided and the sternohyoid muscles are separated.

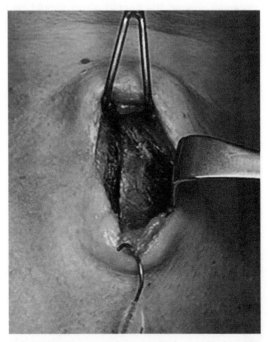

Fig. 4. The sternohyoid muscle is retracted to expose the sternothyroid muscle, which is also retracted.

of tumor anteriorly into the overlying strap musculature. If this is encountered, the surgeon can include a portion of the overlying sternothyroid muscle to ensure a negative margin. Most commonly the sternothyroid muscle is not involved and can be gently lateralized off the thyroid and preserved as the thyroid capsule is exposed (**Fig. 5**).

Attention is now turned to the midline, prelaryngeal region. The pyramidal lobe is identified, traced superiorly, divided superiorly, and reflected inferiorly. The pyramidal lobe may be midline or may extend to either side. Prelaryngeal nodes are removed, and care is taken to not injure the cricothyroid membrane, which is the thinnest point to the airway. Next, the isthmus should be carefully examined and palpated for nodules. The tracheal region is cleared just below the isthmus, and inferior thyroid veins below the isthmus are divided. If no nodules are present, the isthmus is divided in the midline (**Fig. 6**). Pretracheal nodes are assessed and removed as needed. With the isthmus divided, the medial portion of the thyroid can safely be released from the anterior tracheal wall until the lateral extent of the trachea is encountered. This early isthmus division provides helpful mobility and rotational freedom to the specimen for the remainder of the procedure.

Lateral Dissection

Attention is now turned to the lateral border of the thyroid gland. Careful dissection of the superficial loose fascial tissue is dissected off the anterolateral thyroid gland and the gland is gently retracted medially to allow visualization of the carotid sheath, which represents the lateral extent of the dissection. Meticulous dissection is performed over the capsule of the thyroid gland. Care is taken to ensure that all fatty tissue is reflected off the intact capsule of the thyroid gland because parathyroid glands may be hidden within this fatty tissue.[9] Vessels are bipolared or ligated on the capsule of the thyroid to

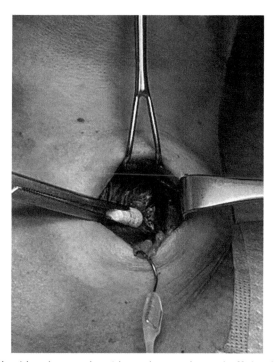

Fig. 5. The sternohyoid and sternothyroid muscles are elevated off the thyroid lobe.

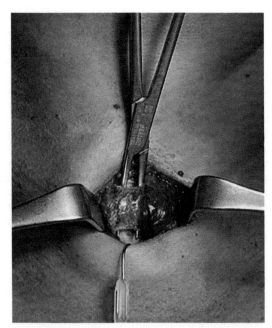

Fig. 6. This isthmus is divided in the midline to expose the anterior trachea and gain mobility to the left thyroid lobe.

prevent potential devascularization of parathyroid glands. The middle thyroid vein is identified, ligated, and divided. The thyroid capsule should seem completely clean of any adjacent tissues with an intact capsule.

Upper Pole Dissection

Attention is now turned to the upper pole. The avascular plane between the medial upper pole and cricothyroid muscle is separated and a clean surgical plane is exposed. The fascia over the cricothyroid muscle is preserved and the dissection stays on the capsule of the thyroid gland in doing so, the upper pole of the thyroid lobe is retracted laterally and inferiorly. This maneuver allows for the identification and preservation of the external branch of the superior laryngeal nerve (EBSLN), which may be stimulated with the nerve monitor probe.[10–12] A visible twitch of the cricothyroid muscle signifies intact stimulation. In most cases, the EBSLN enters the cricothyroid muscle superiorly, but in some cases, it may enter inferiorly and be more vulnerable to injury.[13,14] The superior thyroid artery and vein are now isolated and visualized. A negative nerve stimulation before taking these vessels with no evidence of cricothyroid stimulation is now performed and signifies that it is safe to ligate and divide the superior thyroid artery and vein at their entry point into the thyroid gland (**Figs. 7** and **8**). Vessels should be ligated as close to the thyroid as possible to avoid inadvertently injuring either the EBSLN or the superior parathyroid gland, which might be located just posterior to the superior pedicle. No remnant tissue of the upper pole should be left behind at this part of the dissection (see **Figs. 7** and **8**). With the superior thyroid vasculature bundle separated from the thyroid, the upper pole can now be further rotated inferiorly to expose the posterior surface of the upper pole. At this location, the surgeon should seek to identify and preserve the superior parathyroid gland with its blood supply (**Figs. 9** and **10**). Once identified, the parathyroid gland is gently released from the

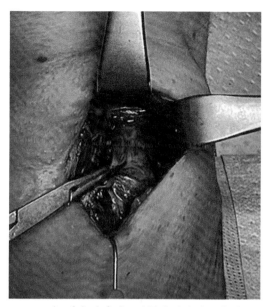

Fig. 7. The superior upper pole of the left thyroid lobe is isolated. The course of the superior laryngeal nerve is determined with the nerve monitor probe and the nerve is protected.

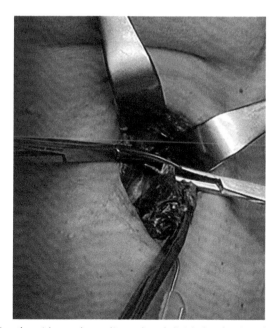

Fig. 8. The superior thyroid vessels are ligated and divided, releasing the superior pole.

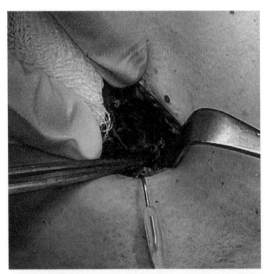

Fig. 9. The gland is retracted medially, and dissection over the thyroid capsule enables the identification and preservation of the superior and inferior parathyroid glands laterally.

capsule of the gland. Minimal manipulation and low power bipolar use ensures preservation of the parathyroid blood supply and gland integrity (**Fig. 11**).

Lower Pole Dissection and Nerve Identification in the Tracheoesophageal Groove

With the upper pole now fully mobilized, attention is again turned laterally and inferiorly to the lower pole of the thyroid lobe. Gentle medial traction on the thyroid gland and pretracheal tissue is placed to allow space along the tracheoesophageal groove. Staying in a plane between the true capsule and investing pretracheal fascia, the fascia is slowly released directly off the thyroid staying as close to the thyroid gland as possible. The inferior parathyroid gland has a highly variable location. Again, meticulous dissection is performed to preserve the parathyroid gland and its blood supply. Only the terminal branches of vessels entering the thyroid gland, distal to the blood

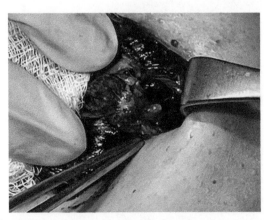

Fig. 10. The superior parathyroid gland is identified on the posterior capsule of the thyroid lobe.

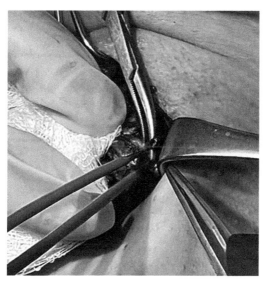

Fig. 11. The parathyroid gland is gently dissected off the thyroid lobe with preservation of its lateral blood supply.

supply to the parathyroid glands, are divided. Ligation of the vessels proximally should be avoided because this will lead to devascularization of the parathyroid gland.[9] Nerve stimulation to identify the RLN should be performed to identify the location of the RLN. When seeking the nerve, a stimulation setting of 2 to 3 mA is useful. Once the nerve is identified, using a lower stimulation of 1 to 1.5 mA for the confirmation of integrity of the nerve is appropriate. The RLN location should be known to the surgeon, either with positive nerve stimulation monitoring and/or visually. The RLN is then protected during continuing dissection on the thyroid capsule to the Berry ligament (**Fig. 12**). The nerve should be treated exceptionally gently with avoidance of unnecessary

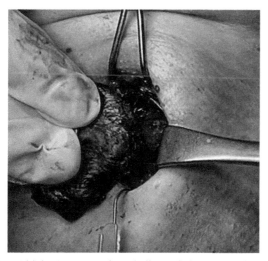

Fig. 12. The left thyroid lobe is retracted medially, and the RLN is identified.

manipulation. Retraction that may pull on the nerve should be avoided. The Bovie electrocautery is avoided completely, and bipolar is used only on low settings when working near the RLN. The RLN integrity is confirmed both anatomically and with stimulation of the nerve (**Fig. 13**). Intact RLN stimulation may lead to amplitudes ranging from 100 to 1000 µV. A drop in the amplitude may signify that the RLN is becoming weak from manipulation and should signal to the surgeon to be gentler with the technique.

If intact RLN stimulation more than 100 µV cannot be achieved, then a checklist should be run to ensure that this is not a problem with the nerve monitor system. The endotracheal tube sensor torque, depth, and tube diameter to establish adequate contact with the glottis should be considered. Grounding leads, cord plugs, and console settings should be evaluated. As a backup control, palpation of twitching of the posterior cricoarytenoid muscle with nerve stimulation can be performed.[15] Find that locating the nerve near its entry into the larynx allows for safe and accurate anatomic location of the nerve while also limiting excessive dissection of the nerve.

With the nerve location and integrity confirmed, dissection is performed to the Berry (suspensory) ligament to release the thyroid lobe medially. The Berry ligament is a dense structure, and sometimes thyroid tissue may be present at the ligament. The RLN should be carefully protected during the division of the Berry ligament.

During dissection of the nerve, the surgeon should be aware that RLN branching may occur. When there is a bifid nerve, the branches may be of very small caliber (1–2 mm) and highly vulnerable to traction injury. Branching of the nerve is most common within 1 cm of its entry point into the cricothyroid membrane.[16] The anterior-most branch is the motor branch; injury to this critical branch leads to vocal cord paresis or paralysis.[16–20] With the nerve in view, the remaining inferior attachments of the thyroid gland to the lateral and anterior tracheal wall inferiorly can now be released.

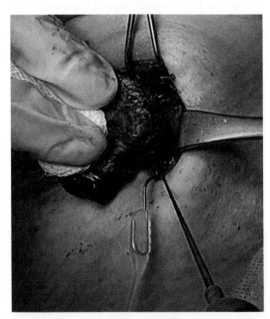

Fig. 13. The left RLN is stimulated with the nerve monitor probe to document its functional integrity.

Removal of the Thyroid Gland

Next, with the gland free from the RLN, the gland is elevated off the remaining attachments through Berry ligament and anterior tracheal wall. Care should be taken to not cause inadvertent injury to the underlying cricothyroid muscle or accidental entry into the trachea. The lobe is now removed and oriented with a silk suture for the pathologist. If a total thyroidectomy is to be performed, attention is turned to the opposite lobe and the steps above are repeated.

Careful inspection of the thyroid gland is performed once it is removed to ensure no parathyroid tissue was inadvertently removed and is found on the thyroid capsule, or under the thyroid capsule in an intrathyroidal location. In this scenario, the parathyroid tissue is removed, frozen section confirmed, minced, and reimplanted into the adjacent sternocleidomastoid muscle. Assessment of the thyroid specimen is now performed to evaluate the lesion removed. The tumor size, texture, capsule status, and potential for extrathyroidal extension are all assessed by the surgeon. The surgical bed is studied for possible lymphadenopathy. A final nerve stimulation of the SLN and RLN is performed, with attention to the signal amplitude obtained.

Layered Closure

The surgical bed is irrigated, and meticulous hemostasis is obtained with the bipolar cautery. The strap muscle fascia is reapproximated in the midline followed by a layered closure of the platysma with inverted knots. Subdermal fine monofilament sutures are placed to reduce incision line tension. Finally, the skin edges are closed in a meticulous fashion with subcuticular, fine, dissolvable monofilament suture. A small adhesive dressing is placed. Drain placement is rarely necessary unless either the thyroid is very large or if a lateral neck dissection is performed.

CLINICS CARE POINTS

- The RLN should always be identified with nerve monitoring and/or visually and carefully preserved with minimal manipulation. Its location should always be known throughout the surgery by the surgeon, although routine dissection and tracing of the RLN may not be necessary. RLN branching leads to more vulnerable anterior division, which may be of small caliber.[18] Traction injury is the most common form of injury to the RLN.

- The superior parathyroid gland is consistently located posterior to the superior pole of the thyroid gland whereas the inferior parathyroid gland has a variable location. Dissection should always be on the thyroid capsule and the tissues with the parathyroid glands should be reflected of the capsule gently with minimal manipulation of the parathyroid glands.

- The EBSLN is at risk during the superior pole dissection. The nerve is the sole motor nerve of the ipsilateral cricothyroid muscle. Injury to the nerve can lead to voice dysfunction with lower voice frequency, lower voice projection, fatigue, and inability to achieve high-frequency sounds.[21] The EBSLN can be preserved reliably using a technique in which the EBSLN is stimulated with the nerve probe to identify its course; a negative stimulation at the superior pole vessels is required before ligation and division of these vessels.

DISCLOSURE

The authors have no disclosures.

REFERENCES

1. Giddings AE. The history of thyroidectomy. J R Soc Med 1998;91(Suppl 33):3–6.

2. Haugen BR, Alexander EK, Bible KC, et al. 2015 American Thyroid Association Management Guidelines for Adult Patients with Thyroid Nodules and Differentiated Thyroid Cancer: The American Thyroid Association Guidelines Task Force on Thyroid Nodules and Differentiated Thyroid Cancer. Thyroid 2016;26(1):1–133.

3. Patel KN, Yip L, Lubitz CC, et al. The American Association of Endocrine Surgeons Guidelines for the Definitive Surgical Management of Thyroid Disease in Adults. Ann Surg 2020;271(3):e21–93.

4. Stojadinovic A, Shoup M, Nissan A, et al. Recurrent differentiated thyroid carcinoma: biological implications of age, method of detection, and site and extent of recurrence. Ann Surg Oncol 2002;9(8):789–98.

5. Nixon IJ, Shaha AR, Patel SG. Surgical diagnosis: frozen section and the extent of surgery. Otolaryngol Clin 2014;47(4):519–28.

6. Matsuura D, Yuan A, Harris V, et al. Surgical Management of Low-/Intermediate-Risk Node Negative Thyroid Cancer: A Single-Institution Study Using Propensity Matching Analysis to Compare Thyroid Lobectomy and Total Thyroidectomy. Thyroid 2022;32(1):28–36.

7. Shah JP, Patel SG, Singh B, et al. Jatin Shah's head and neck surgery and oncology. 5th edition. New York, NY: Elsevier; 2020.

8. Sinos G, Sakorafas GH. Pyramidal lobe of the thyroid: anatomical considerations of importance in thyroid cancer surgery. Oncol Res Treat 2015;38(6):309–10.

9. Uslu A, Okut G, Tercan IC, et al. Anatomical distribution and number of parathyroid glands, and parathyroid function, after total parathyroidectomy and bilateral cervical thymectomy. Medicine (Baltim) 2019;98(23):e15926.

10. Cheruiyot I, Kipkorir V, Henry BM, et al. Surgical anatomy of the external branch of the superior laryngeal nerve: a systematic review and meta-analysis. Langenbeck's Arch Surg 2018;403(7):811–23.

11. Barczyński M, Randolph GW, Cernea CR, et al. External branch of the superior laryngeal nerve monitoring during thyroid and parathyroid surgery: International Neural Monitoring Study Group standards guideline statement. Laryngoscope 2013;123(Suppl 4):S1–14.

12. Sulica L. The superior laryngeal nerve: function and dysfunction. Otolaryngol Clin 2004;37(1):183–201.

13. Potenza AS, Araujo Filho VJF, Cernea CR. Injury of the external branch of the superior laryngeal nerve in thyroid surgery. Gland Surg 2017;6(5):552–62.

14. Kambic V, Zargi M, Radsel Z. Topographic anatomy of the external branch of the superior laryngeal nerve. Its importance in head and neck surgery. J Laryngol Otol 1984;98(11):1121–4.

15. Shindo M, Chheda NN. Incidence of vocal cord paralysis with and without recurrent laryngeal nerve monitoring during thyroidectomy. Arch Otolaryngol Head Neck Surg 2007;133(5):481–5.

16. Henry BM, Vikse J, Graves MJ, et al. Extralaryngeal branching of the recurrent laryngeal nerve: a meta-analysis of 28,387 nerves. Langenbeck's Arch Surg 2016;401(7):913–23.

17. Shindo ML, Wu JC, Park EE. Surgical anatomy of the recurrent laryngeal nerve revisited. Otolaryngol Head Neck Surg 2005;133(4):514–9.

18. Randolph GW, Dralle H. International Intraoperative Monitoring Study Group, et al. Electrophysiologic recurrent laryngeal nerve monitoring during thyroid and parathyroid surgery: international standards guideline statement. Laryngoscope 2011;121(Suppl 1):S1–16.

19. Gür EO, Haciyanli M, Karaisli S, et al. Intraoperative nerve monitoring during thyroidectomy: evaluation of signal loss, prognostic value and surgical strategy. Ann R Coll Surg Engl 2019;101(8):589–95.
20. Kovatch KJ, Reyes-Gastelum D, Hughes DT, et al. Assessment of Voice Outcomes Following Surgery for Thyroid Cancer. JAMA Otolaryngol Head Neck Surg 2019;145(9):823–9.
21. Henry LR, Solomon NP, Howard R, et al. The functional impact on voice of sternothyroid muscle division during thyroidectomy. Ann Surg Oncol 2008;15(7): 2027–33.

Surgical Management of Substernal Thyroid Goiters

Amanda J. Bastien, MD[a,b], Allen S. Ho, MD[a,b],*

KEYWORDS

- Multinodular thyroid goiter • Substernal thyroid goiter • Thyroidectomy • Sternotomy

KEY POINTS

- Multidisciplinary coordination with endocrinology, otolaryngology-head and neck surgery, anesthesia, and thoracic surgery is essential for determining the optimal management of substernal thyroid goiter.
- Preoperative workup includes cross-sectional imaging of the neck and chest (ie, computed tomography or magnetic resonance imaging), which characterizes the gland and its relationship to vital structures such as the esophagus, trachea, and great vessels.
- Surgery for substernal thyroid goiter is typically recommended for compressive symptoms, suspicion for malignancy, and excessive hyperthyroidism.
- The combined cervical-thoracic approach with sternotomy confers greater access for resection but poses greater risk of intraoperative complications and longer postoperative rehabilitation.

INTRODUCTION

The substernal thyroid goiter was first described in the literature by Haller in 1749, yet it was not until 1820 when its resection was first reported by Klein.[1,2] Such a condition can present with interdisciplinary surgical challenges due to anatomic constraints, anesthesia considerations, and critical adjacent structures. Substernal goiters further inhabit a space associated with swallowing and breathing. In this article, the surgical management of substernal thyroid glands will be discussed in detail including preoperative workup, the cervical approach, the combined cervical-thoracic approach, and complications.

DISCUSSION
Anatomy

A substernal goiter, or retrosternal goiter, occurs when thyroid tissue descends into the mediastinum through the thoracic inlet. Typically, the thyroid grows anteriorly

[a] Division of Otolaryngology–Head and Neck Surgery, Department of Surgery, Cedars-Sinai Medical Center, Los Angeles, CA, USA; [b] Samuel Oschin Comprehensive Cancer Institute, Cedars-Sinai Medical Center, Los Angeles, CA, USA
* Corresponding author. 8631 West 3rd Street, #915E, Los Angeles, CA 90048.
E-mail address: Allen.Ho@cshs.org

Otolaryngol Clin N Am 57 (2024) 39–52
https://doi.org/10.1016/j.otc.2023.07.008
0030-6665/24/© 2023 Elsevier Inc. All rights reserved.

oto.theclinics.com

and/or laterally during aberrant growth. Most goiters are located in the anterior mediastinum (85%).[3,4]

To be considered a true substernal goiter, more than 50% of the thyroid tissue is located below the sternal notch according to Katilic, Grillo, and Wang.[5] Other definitions for substernal thyroid in the literature include thyroid tissue located 3 cm below the sternal notch or thyroid tissue that has descended below the fourth thoracic vertebra.[6–9] Diameter and goiter weight have both been used in the literature to quantify thyroid enlargement. The average weight (grams) of a substernal goiter is 104 g (ranging from 25 to 357 g), and a diameter ranging from 5 cm to 19 cm.[10] Extension of thyroid tissue into the mediastinum is overall uncommon, seen in less than 5% of patients undergoing thyroidectomy.[11]

The presence of distinct ectopic thyroid tissue in the chest is rare, making up only 2% of all substernal goiters.[12] In this subset of mediastinal goiters, the blood supply originates from the mediastinum, which can include the aorta, subclavian, internal mammary, thyrocervical trunk, and the innominate vessels. In some cases, a cervical goiter descends into the mediastinum and then can lose its continuity with thyroid tissue. It may also be marginally attached with fascial extension and can be mistaken for ectopic thyroid tissue.

Substernal goiters are adenomatous and usually benign but carcinoma has been identified in 2% to 19% of patients.[11] Substernal goiters are more commonly diagnosed in patients aged older than 50 years and are 4 times more common in women.[13] Goiter development has been associated with smoking history, autoimmune thyroid diseases, iodine deficiency, and malignancy.[13] Earlier family and twin studies have indicated a genetic predisposition to goiter development with autosomal dominant inheritance pattern with locus heterogeneity.[14,15] Due to their role in thyroid physiology and hormone production, multiple genes (eg, TG, TSHR, TSHB, and SLC5A5) have been found to be associated with familial goiter.[16–18] Goiter development is complex and the interplay of poorly described environmental factors interacting with a genetic predisposition is likely to lead to development and growth.[18]

Preoperative Evaluation

It is important to note a wide range of substernal thyroid goiter patients (15%–50%) are asymptomatic.[6] Nonetheless, patients may complain of local obstructive or compressive symptoms that include exertional dyspnea, chocking sensation, dysphagia, cough, and stridor. Liddy and colleagues published a series in which shortness of breath and/or dysphagia affected approximately 50% of patients.[19] In this series, there was a positive correlation between thyroid size and globus sensation, as well as an association between dysphagia and the presence of esophageal compression and deviation. There was also a significant relationship between the presence of shortness of breath and objective CT (computerized tomography) radiographic findings of tracheal compression. Interestingly, no correlation was observed with thyroid size and dysphagia, local discomfort, and voice changes.[19] In cases in which there is compression of the trachea by extracervical thyroid tissue, stridor may be audible. Thyroid dysfunction, whether hyperthyroidism or hypothyroidism, can occur with substernal goiter, and related symptoms should be discussed when reviewing the patient history.

On physical examination, the thyroid should be palpated to examine for mobility, deviation, or exacerbation of symptoms on deep pressure. Pemberton sign (ie, facial congestion and cyanosis when elevating arms due to obstruction of superior vena cava return) should be assessed during the physical examination.[20] These physical changes in the patient suggest compression or "corking" of the thyroid at the thoracic inlet.

An endocrinology consult is important as part of the comprehensive workup and will typically include thyroid function tests. Flexible fiberoptic laryngoscopy is also helpful to assess the airway for deviation, edema, vocal cord paralysis, and anesthesia planning on intubation. Michel and colleagues report hoarseness was apparent in 26% preoperative patients with substernal goiter but only 3% had vocal cord paralysis on laryngeal examination preoperatively.[21,22] The use of fine-needle aspiration (FNA) is helpful in evaluating thyroid nodules in cervical goiters for malignancy but its utility is limited in substernal goiters due to poor access to the mediastinum.[22,23] FNA should still be performed for sonographically suspicious nodules in the cervical goiter to assess malignancy risk, which may change the nature of the operation.

The most important imaging modality is CT of the neck and chest. Imaging is especially helpful to assess for the displacement of the trachea, esophagus, and regional vessels.[21] Preoperative CT with the patient's neck in extension has been reported as valuable in surgical planning, including whether to consent for sternotomy.[7,24] Depending on the institution, some CT neck protocols cover the upper third of the chest beyond the aorta and are sufficient for capturing substernal goiters in their entirety. In comparison, many CT chest protocols will by themselves fail to completely capture the superior extent of thyroid goiters.

As an alternative, MRI (magnetic resonance imaging) can provide more comprehensive soft tissue detail, whether there is invasion of vascular structures, and can be useful for patients with iodine contrast allergies who need to minimize radiation exposure. Although more than half of cases with substernal extension can be detected on whole body radionuclide scans, such imaging modalities have poor anatomic delineation and resolution compared with MRI/CT and are not routinely used.[5]

Contrast, whether it be iodine for CT or gadolinium for MRI, is not mandatory but has been historically underappreciated for surgical planning. Characterization of the goiter's abutment or encasement of vasculature (ie, innominate vessels, the thyrocervical trunk, and the common carotid arteries) can determine the need to prepare for blood products, thoracic surgery assistance, or even sternotomy approaches (**Fig. 1**). Visualization of the carotid sheath further helps with preoperatively estimating localization of the recurrent laryngeal nerve (RLN) and gauging risk for traction injury. As such, we routinely recommend contrast for substernal goiters.

Management

A substernal goiter alone, with or without symptoms, can be an indication for intervention, given likelihood of progression.[25] Surgery is also recommended when there is suspicion for malignancy or excessive hyperthyroidism.[26]

Radioactive Iodine and Levothyroxine Suppression

An important consideration before surgery is to assess whether the patient can tolerate general anesthesia. Patients deemed at high risk for anesthesia are contraindicated for substernal thyroidectomy. For all patients with a substernal goiter, there is a possibility for total obstruction of the distal trachea after induction. In patients who medically cannot undergo anesthesia due to comorbidities cases, especially in the absence of goiter-related symptoms, conservative management or radioiodine treatment is usually preferred.[23] In cases of dispersed, multifocal recurrence where revision thyroidectomy cannot excise all components, radioactive iodine (RAI) after revision thyroidectomy has achieved a gross total resection may be considered to prevent further recurrence.

In general, most agree that medical treatment (ie, thyroxine suppression or RAI) are not durable options for substernal goiters.[5] A substernal goiter is difficult to monitor on

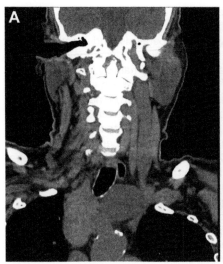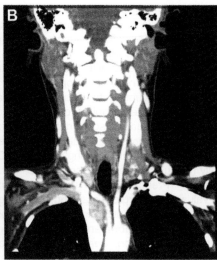

Fig. 1. Comparative use of CT neck imaging with or without contrast. (*A*) CT neck without contrast in a 66-year-old man with papillary thyroid carcinoma (PTC) and mediastinal/level 7 metastatic lymph nodes (LN). The relationship of the 2 metastatic LN to the innominate vessels is ambiguous. (*B*). CT neck with contrast in a 46-year-old woman with PTC and mediastinal/level 7 LN inferior to the innominate artery.

physical examination and likely to progress in size. Although there is evidence that RAI can reduce the goiter volume by 40% to 60%, this is more likely to occur in younger patients, smaller sized goiters, and cervical goiters.[27,28] The use of radioiodine therapy may further induce acute inflammation and swelling of the gland, carrying meaningful risk for potential for airway obstruction.

The use of thyroid hormone suppressive therapy remains controversial. Berghout and colleagues showed a 25% or greater goiter volume reduction using thyroxine suppression in a randomized control trial in 58% of patients with goiter. However, after stopping suppression therapy, the goiters regrew.[29] It seems some goiters respond, whereas others grow despite thyroid suppressive therapy, and the consensus is that it is ineffective in most cases. Undesirable side effects of indefinite suppressive therapy are significant which include bone demineralization and cardiac arrythmias.[30,31]

Total Thyroidectomy Versus Lobectomy

Numerous factors should be considered when determining the extent of surgery. For bilateral benign thyroid goiter, a total thyroidectomy should be performed. This is due to lower risk of recurrent goiter over time (0%–0.5%) versus greater than 10% in subtotal thyroidectomy.[23] A total thyroidectomy is also indicated in cases of hyperthyroidism or concern for malignancy.[32]

Lobectomy (also known as hemithyroidectomy) may confer unique advantages and be indicated in particular situations. In the case of a unilateral goiter, a lobectomy can be performed with low recurrence rates and potentially obviate lifelong thyroid hormone replacement.[23]

According to Bauer and colleagues, hemithyroidectomy had a lower complication rate (8% vs 26%, $P < .001$) but there was no difference in the rate of permanent complications (0.2% vs 1%, $P = .133$).[33] Importantly, thyroid hormone replacement was needed in only 19% of substernal goiter patients who underwent a lobectomy.[33]

Cervical Versus Combined Cervical-Thoracic Approach

When deciding to do a cervical versus combined cervical-thoracic approach (partial sternotomy or full sternotomy), it is important for patients and surgeons to honestly weigh the risks and benefits. CT or MRI scans can assist in determining if the facial planes around the gland are present. This helps inform the surgeon whether the gland may be mobilized through the thoracic inlet, or if an extended approach by sternotomy will be warranted.[23]

Patients who avoid sternotomy rehabilitate faster postoperatively ($P = .028$): postoperative discharge is 1.79 ± 1.59 for cervical approach versus 3.14 ± 0.9 days with combined approach requiring a sternotomy.[34–36] The combined cervical-thoracic approach poses more risk of intraoperative complications, in addition to a longer postoperative recovery. In assessing long-term complications and outcomes, patients who underwent a combined approach still had excellent outcomes making a sternotomy a safe procedure when performed by experienced surgeons.[34]

A lesion requiring a sternotomy for complete resection is shown in **Fig. 2**. However, such an approach for substernal goiter is estimated to be needed in only 2% of cases.[23] In contrast, Monchik and colleagues reported that 27 of 94 patients identified on CT with a mediastinal thyroid mass (29% of patients) required a thoracic approach for substernal thyroid (21 partial sternotomies, 5 full sternotomies, and 1 right posterolateral thoracotomy). It is essential to note that 15 out of 27 patients (56% of thoracic approach cases) in this study were for malignant thyroid pathologic condition.[37] Altogether, thyroid surgeons must gain familiarity with thoracic approaches, including when to refer to thoracic surgery for preoperative consultation, especially for cancer.

For substernal goiters, it is always valuable to discuss the case with a thoracic surgeon beforehand and to prep the chest and drape in case the thoracic access is needed for either (1) thyroid retrieval or (2) inaccessible bleeding. This should be

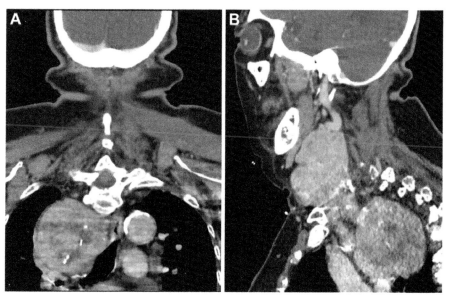

Fig. 2. Substernal thyroid variants illustrated on CT neck imaging. Both cases necessitate consideration of sternotomy for appropriate access. (*A*). Ectopic thyroid issue, distinct from the thyroid gland. (*B*) Thyroid goiter with extension to the posterior mediastinum.

included in preoperative counseling with the patient. A formal consult with thoracic surgery is recommended if the likelihood of a sternotomy is considered high.

Items to consider preoperatively that favor sternotomy include if the substernal goiter is larger than the thoracic inlet, located in the posterior mediastinum, close proximity to the carina, encasement or compression of critical vessels (eg, innominate vessels, aortic arch, superior vena cava), trachea and esophagus deviation or narrowing, and recurrent goiter.[22] Morselization to decrease goiter size and assist in the piecemeal delivery of the gland has been reported. This technique was first described by Kocher in 1889 and was subsequently popularized by Lahey in 1945. This technique is not routinely recommended due to the high risk of bleeding, retraction of remnant thyroid tissue deeper into the chest and potential cancer dissemination.[19]

Partial Versus Full Sternotomy

When extracervical access is indicated, the extent of sternotomy must weigh proper surgical access with potentially longer patient recovery as considerations (**Table 1**). If the substernal goiter is in the anterior mediastinum but on imaging seems larger than the thoracic inlet or adhered to important structures, a partial sternotomy is a useful approach for resection for goiters located superior or at the level of the aortic arch. The patient should be positioned similarly to a cervical goiter with a shoulder roll. It is important to ensure the shoulder roll is located at the scapulae to ensure neck extension; this maneuver shifts the carina more anteriorly. Even when sternotomy is planned, the cervical part of the goiter is addressed first and then attention should be turned to the substernal portion using a T-shaped skin incision (extending to below the angle of Louis). If the patient presents with superior vena cava syndrome, addressing the substernal portion allows for venous pressure reduction and decreases the risk of bleeding during cervical dissection.[38] After incision, the sternal notch is exposed and using electrocautery and blunt dissection, the posterior fascial plane is removed posteriorly. When maneuvering near the posterior sternal notch, gentle manipulation should mobilize the innominate vein and pleura away from the posterior sternum. The upper part of the sternum is opened and retracted laterally to reveal the upper mediastinum, thereby giving access the trachea, esophagus, and innominate vein and artery. The mediastinal portion of the substernal goiter can then be accessed more freely.

A complete sternotomy includes an incision extending from the sternal notch to the xiphoid tip and confers both the greatest exposure to the anterior mediastinum and easier access to the posterior mediastinum (**Fig. 3**). The partial or full median sternotomy is closed with heavy-gauge stainless steel wires in the sternum (**Fig. 4**). Postoperative complications are the same as partial sternotomy, which include bleeding due to injury to vasculature or other important structures, wound infection, sternal dehiscence, mediastinitis, and pneumothorax. Pericardial injury and heart injury although extremely rare may occur while performing a full sternotomy.

Patients who undergo a sternal split or complete sternotomy should have a chest radiograph postoperatively to assess the pleural space to ensure no effusion or pneumothorax. If a substantial pneumothorax or effusion is present, it should be drained with a thoracostomy tube. If there is robust bloody output, this should raise concern for hemorrhage and returning for operative evaluation should be considered.

In comparing patients who underwent partial versus full sternotomy, patients treated with partial upper sternotomy had better pulmonary function and reduced pain compared with patients treated with complete sternotomy.[39] The same number of complications was observed between the two approaches, but longer hospital and ICU stays were associated with those who had full sternotomy procedures.[39]

Table 1
Common sternotomy techniques, indications, and considerations

Type of Sternotomy	Technique	Indication	Considerations
Partial	Incision is made vertically from the midportion of the neck incision to the manubriosternal junction	• No fascial plane visible on CT/MRI • Goiter larger than thoracic inlet • Close proximity to carina and vessels • Trachea or esophagus deviation/narrowing	• Better pulmonary function than full sternotomy • Similar complication rate to full sternotomy
Full	Incision is taken down to the xiphoid process	• Goiter extends to posterior mediastinum • Goiter extends to aortic arch • Need for greater exposure; eg, neoplasms that may invade the great vessels or distal airway	• Better visualization than neck incision • More pain than neck incision • Longer hospital stay

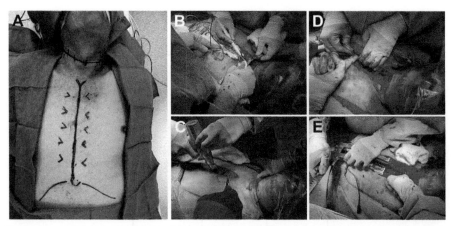

Fig. 3. Planned full sternotomy incision in a patient with large mediastinal extension of substernal goiter. (*A*) Preoperative marking with the shoulder roll under scapulae, marking the sternal notch superiorly and the xiphoid inferiorly. (*B*) Connection of sternotomy incision to the thyroidectomy incision. (*C*) Splitting of sternum with reciprocating sternal saw. (*D*) Bone wax applied to the sternum. (*E*) Mediastinal exposure with Finochietto retractor/rib spreader.

Technical Considerations for Thyroidectomy

Because substernal goiter is often associated with distorted anatomy, proper access is fundamental to the operation. A large apron or collar incision is necessary to achieve appropriate exposure. Sectioning the deep strap musculature (ie, the sternothyroid

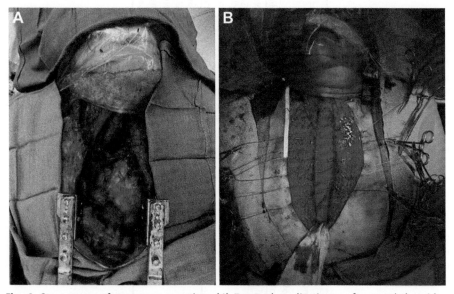

Fig. 4. Sternotomy after cancer resection. (*A*) Exposed mediastinum after total thyroidectomy and level 6/7 mediastinal node dissection, with sternal retractor in place. (*B*) Heavy-gauge stainless steel sternal wires placed for closure.

muscle) and partially incising the medial border of the sternocleidomastoid muscle at the clavicle can further widen access, although this is not always necessary. Dissection of the carotid sheath can also be helpful: the relationship of the great vessels with the goiter as they enter the mediastinum is important for anticipating involvement of innominate vessels or the aortic arch, and following the vagus nerve inferiorly may better triangulate the location of the RLN (either through tracing the vagus or through intermittent stimulation with nerve monitoring). For extensive superior goiter extent, meticulous control of engorged superior thyroid vessels is necessary to avoid retraction and problematic bleeding. Similarly, protecting the superior laryngeal nerve should also not be underestimated because there is likely a higher risk of injury from anatomic distortion.

During cases where a total thyroidectomy is performed, it may be useful to first free the smaller thyroid lobe or divide the 2 lobes at the midline to facilitate substernal mobilization. It also is helpful in the identification process of the RLN and the parathyroid glands. Preservation of the parathyroid glands is of great importance and should be identified before goiter excision. It is important to be aware that the position of the RLN can be variable in cases of goiters.

To facilitate cervical delivery of substernal goiter, the use of blunt manual dissection can be highly effective by adding tactile feedback to a potentially blind space. This presumes the RLN has been identified, so as to avoid inadvertent traction injury. Blunt-tipped bipolar energy devices such as the small-jaw Ligasure are also helpful for cauterizing deep mediastinal tissue bands or vessels that tether the thyroid. Using larger grasping clamps often found in the thoracic tray (ie, Lahey traction forceps) and at multiple points along the goiter may help avoid unnecessary avulsion of tissue while hoisting the goiter superiorly for safer, easier dissection.

Recurrent Laryngeal Nerve Pearls

The cricothyroid junction and the inferior thyroid artery can be used as helpful landmarks to assist in the identification of the nerve when anatomy may be distorted. The nerves passes posterior to the cricothyroid joint as it enters the larynx and commonly courses deep to the inferior thyroid artery. The use of intraoperative neural monitoring of the RLN has been widely used to avoid nerve injury during the thyroidectomy portion.[40,41] The vagus nerve can be identified while completing the carotid sheath dissection and can be stimulated during the surgery to ensure the nerve is intact during maneuvers that may cause neural stretch. Such potential inadvertent traction may lead some to use continuous intraoperative nerve monitoring: the real-time feedback on the RLN functional state helps alert surgeons during potentially blind maneuvers from mediastinal tissue manipulation.

It is important to note that substernal goiter can substantially alter the expected course and appearance of the RLN. Approximately 15% to 20% of substernal goiters have been found to have RLNs that are splayed, entrapped, or fixed to the goiter, such that blind delivery of the thyroid gland through the skin or significant traction could lead to injury.[7] Especially in posterior mediastinal goiters (**Fig. 5**), thyroid tissue may run deep to the RLN, leading to superficial displacement and a ventrally positioned nerve. Finally, a nerve passively stretched over time by a large goiter may seem deceptively thin, similar in appearance to fascial band attachments. As such, meticulous capsular dissection along the thyroid gland with nerve stimulation before any cautery is necessary to avoid accidental transection. Identification of the RLN, using the vague nerve to help predict its location, is strongly recommended if possible before delivering the goiter.

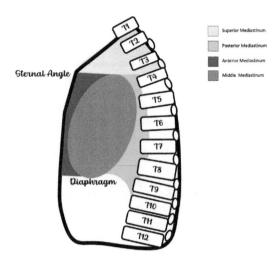

Fig. 5. The mediastinum regions and associated borders. About 85% of substernal thyroid goiters are in the anterior mediastinum.

Parathyroid Gland Pearls

During surgery, it is helpful to identify the inferior thyroid artery, ligating it directly on the thyroid capsule. This maneuver helps preserve parathyroid tissue and its blood supply. The distal inferior thyroid artery should only be taken after the RLN is identified. The RLN commonly runs anterior to the inferior thyroid artery on the right side, and often runs posterior to the inferior thyroid artery on the left side.[42] The location of the inferior parathyroids is more variable than that of superior parathyroid glands.[42] It is important to inspect the thyroid gland after delivery to ensure there are no capsular parathyroids; if located, these glands should be dissected free before removal or if found after delivery reimplanted.

Complications

Patients with retrosternal goiters are more likely to have transient and, in some cases, permanent RLN injury and permanent hypoparathyroidism after surgery compared with patients with cervical goiters.[43,44] Testini and colleagues report 3.2% of patients had transient unilateral RLN palsy after cervical thyroidectomy versus 5.5% in patients who had a total thyroidectomy for a substernal goiter.[43] Tracheobronchial fistula or sternotomy dehiscence is a major complication contributing to reported patient mortalities but overall mortality is rare.[45] Thyroid cancer and compression symptoms are also related to poorer outcomes.[23,45]

The occurrence of a hemorrhage usually occurs within the first 8 hours after surgery and can be a devastating complication due to laryngeal edema and airway obstruction.[28] The incidence of hemorrhage has been reported to be 4.2%.[46] The use of a Jackson-Pratt drain can help recognize active or developing hemorrhage. Other rare complications include infection, pneumothorax, and the need for tracheostomy.

Tracheomalacia

It is noteworthy to mention tracheomalacia as a concern often mentioned by anesthesiology in substernal thyroid goiter. This phenomenon is characterized by prolapse of floppy tracheal rings, narrowing the trachea lumen. The underlying pathophysiology for tracheomalacia can be congenital due to cartilage immaturity, observed more in the pediatric population with congenital anomalies or in a premature state. Tracheomalacia can also be acquired, potentially resulting from goiter mass effect or chronic infection. The incidence of this condition after thyroidectomy in mature adults is rare and contested (0%–5.3%),[23] leading some to question whether it truly exists. Regardless, the detection of tracheomalacia should be straightforward to diagnose after thyroidectomy, both by the surgeon (by intraoperative palpation or visualization after thyroidectomy) and the anesthesiologist (by decreased tidal volumes). Treatment may necessitate prolonged intubation, close observation after extubation with a bougie, or tracheostomy.

SUMMARY

Patients with a substernal thyroid goiter is best managed by a multidisciplinary team, which encompasses endocrinology, otolaryngology-head and neck surgery, anesthesia, and thoracic surgery. Substernal thyroid goiters may not always confer symptoms but surgery is often recommended. The vast majority of substernal goiters can be removed using a transcervical incision. Complications associated with substernal goiters are higher compared with cervical goiters. With careful planning and an experienced team, a safe and successful operation can nonetheless be achieved.

CLINICS CARE POINTS

- Management of substernal thyroid goiter warrants thoughtful preoperative counseling and the expertise of a multidisciplinary team.

- Preoperative imaging greatly facilitates surgical planning and determining the need for sternotomy.

- Surgical management is the recommended treatment of symptomatic substernal thyroid goiters. The need for a combined cervical approach to the mediastinum is rare.

- Intraoperative nerve monitoring can be helpful, given that RLN anatomy can be displaced, splayed, and distorted by the goiter.

- Complications are higher in patients with substernal goiters compared with cervical goiters. Surgical management should be performed by experienced surgical teams.

- Goiters with extension into the posterior mediastinum often displace the RLN ventrally. Particular care should be taken to avoid traction or avulsion injuries.

DISCLOSURE

The authors have no conflicts of interest relevant to this article to disclose.

REFERENCES

1. Von Haller A. Disputationes anatomicae selectae: ill., Graph. Darst. Vandenhoeck; 1747.
2. Klein F. Veber die Austrotting verschiedener geschwulste, besonders jener der Ohrspercheldruse und der Schiddruse; Aussachalung der Schilddruse. J Chir Augenlleilk 1820;12:106–13.
3. Shahian DM, Rossi RL. Posterior mediastinal goiter. Chest 1988;94(3):599–602.
4. Cho HT, Cohen JP, Som ML. Management of Substernal and Intrathoracic Goiters. Otolaryngol Neck Surg 1986;94(3):282–7.

5. Wang L-S. Surgical management of a substernal goiter. Formos J Surg 2012; 45(2):41–4.
6. Katlic MR, Wang C, Grillo HC. Substernal Goiter. Ann Thorac Surg 1985;39(4): 391–9.
7. Coskun A, Yildirim M, Erkan N. Substernal goiter: when is a sternotomy required? Int Surg 2014;99(4):419–25.
8. Flati G, De Giacomo T, Porowska B, et al. Surgical management of substernal goitres. When is sternotomy inevitable? Clin Ter 2005;156(5):191–5.
9. Rodriguez JM, Hernandez Q, Piñero A, et al. Substernal goiter: clinical experience of 72 cases. Ann Otol Rhinol Laryngol 1999;108(5):501–4.
10. Katlic MR, Grillo HC, Wang CA. Substernal goiter. Analysis of 80 patients from Massachusetts General Hospital. Am J Surg 1985;149(2):283–7.
11. Chávez Tostado KV, Velázquez-Fernandez D, Chapa M, et al. Substernal Goiter: Correlation between Grade and Surgical Approach. Am Surg 2018;84(2):262–6.
12. Patel KN, Yip L, Lubitz CC, et al. The American Association of Endocrine Surgeons Guidelines for the Definitive Surgical Management of Thyroid Disease in Adults. Ann Surg 2020;271(3):e21–93.
13. Chen AY, Bernet VJ, Carty SE, et al. American Thyroid Association Statement on Optimal Surgical Management of Goiter. Thyroid 2014;24(2):181–9.
14. Bignell GR, Canzian F, Shayeghi M, et al. Familial nontoxic multinodular thyroid goiter locus maps to chromosome 14q but does not account for familial nonmedullary thyroid cancer. Am J Hum Genet 1997;61(5):1123–30.
15. Neumann S, Willgerodt H, Ackermann F, et al. Linkage of familial euthyroid goiter to the multinodular goiter-1 locus and exclusion of the candidate genes thyroglobulin, thyroperoxidase, and Na+/I- symporter. J Clin Endocrinol Metab 1999;84(10):3750–6.
16. Krohn K, Führer D, Bayer Y, et al. Molecular pathogenesis of euthyroid and toxic multinodular goiter. Endocr Rev 2005;26(4):504–24.
17. Park SM, Chatterjee VKK. Genetics of congenital hypothyroidism. J Med Genet 2005;42(5):379–89.
18. Yan J, Takahashi T, Ohura T, et al. Combined linkage analysis and exome sequencing identifies novel genes for familial goiter. J Hum Genet 2013;58(6): 366–77.
19. Liddy W, Netterville JL, Soylu S, et al. Surgery of cervical and substernal goiter. In: Surgery of the thyroid and parathyroid glands. Elsevier; 2021. p. 53–69.e6. https://doi.org/10.1016/B978-0-323-66127-0.00006-5.
20. Basaria S, Salvatori R. Pemberton's Sign. N Engl J Med 2004;350(13):1338.
21. Michel LA. Surgery of substernal goiter. Acta Oto-Rhino-Laryngol Belg 1987; 41(5):863–80.
22. Michel LA, Bradpiece HA. Surgical management of substernal goitre. Br J Surg 1988;75(6):565–9.
23. Nixon IJ, Simo R. The neoplastic goitre. Curr Opin Otolaryngol Head Neck Surg 2013;21(2):143–9.
24. Yano T, Okada T, Sato H, et al. Preoperative Evaluation of Substernal Goiter by Computed Tomography in the Extended Neck Position. Case Rep Oncol 2021; 14(3):1353–8.
25. Allo MD, Thompson NW. Rationale for the operative management of substernal goiters. Surgery 1983;94(6):969–77.
26. Fortuny JV, Guigard S, Karenovics W, et al. Surgery of the thyroid: recent developments and perspective. Swiss Med Wkly 2015;145:w14144.

27. Bonnema SJ, Fast S, Nielsen VE, et al. Serum thyroxine and age–rather than thyroid volume and serum TSH–are determinants of the thyroid radioiodine uptake in patients with nodular goiter. J Endocrinol Invest 2011;34(3):e52–7.
28. Bonnema SJ, Knudsen DU, Bertelsen H, et al. Does radioiodine therapy have an equal effect on substernal and cervical goiter volumes? Evaluation by magnetic resonance imaging. Thyroid 2002;12(4):313–7.
29. Berghout A, Wiersinga WM, Drexhage HA, et al. Comparison of placebo with L-thyroxine alone or with carbimazole for treatment of sporadic non-toxic goitre. Lancet Lond Engl 1990;336(8709):193–7.
30. Uzzan B, Campos J, Cucherat M, et al. Effects on bone mass of long term treatment with thyroid hormones: a meta-analysis. J Clin Endocrinol Metab 1996; 81(12):4278–89.
31. Rieu M, Bekka S, Sambor B, et al. Prevalence of subclinical hyperthyroidism and relationship between thyroid hormonal status and thyroid ultrasonographic parameters in patients with non-toxic nodular goitre. Clin Endocrinol 1993;39(1): 67–71.
32. Haugen BR, Alexander EK, Bible KC, et al. 2015 American Thyroid Association Management Guidelines for Adult Patients with Thyroid Nodules and Differentiated Thyroid Cancer: The American Thyroid Association Guidelines Task Force on Thyroid Nodules and Differentiated Thyroid Cancer. Thyroid 2016;26(1):1–133.
33. Bauer PS, Murray S, Clark N, et al. Unilateral thyroidectomy for the treatment of benign multinodular goiter. J Surg Res 2013;184(1):514–8.
34. Nankee L, Chen H, Schneider DF, et al. Substernal goiter: when is a sternotomy required? J Surg Res 2015;199(1):121–5.
35. Kilic D, Findikcioglu A, Ekici Y, et al. When is transthoracic approach indicated in retrosternal goiters? Ann Thorac Cardiovasc Surg 2011;17(3):250–3.
36. Batori M, Chatelou E, Straniero A, et al. Substernal goiters. Eur Rev Med Pharmacol Sci 2005;9(6):355–9.
37. Monchik JM, Materazzi G. The necessity for a thoracic approach in thyroid surgery. Arch Surg Chic Ill 1960 2000;135(4):467–71, discussion 471-472.
38. Anonymous, Richer SL, Lang BHH, Lo CY, et al. Substernal goiter. In: Terris DJ, Duke WS, editors. Thyroid and parathyroid diseases. Medical and surgical management. 2nd edition. New York: Thieme Publishers; 2016. p. 132–9.
39. Candaele S, Herijgers P, Demeyere R, et al. Chest pain after partial upper versus complete sternotomy for aortic valve surgery. Acta Cardiol 2003;58(1):17–21.
40. Liddy W, Wu C-W, Dionigi G, et al. Varied Recurrent Laryngeal Nerve Course Is Associated with Increased Risk of Nerve Dysfunction During Thyroidectomy: Results of the Surgical Anatomy of the Recurrent Laryngeal Nerve in Thyroid Surgery Study, an International Multicenter Prospective Anatomic and Electrophysiologic Study of 1000 Monitored Nerves at Risk from the International Neural Monitoring Study Group. Thyroid 2021;31(11):1730–40.
41. Gür EO, Haciyanli M, Karaisli S, et al. Intraoperative nerve monitoring during thyroidectomy: evaluation of signal loss, prognostic value and surgical strategy. Ann R Coll Surg Engl 2019;101(8):589–95.
42. Noussios G, Chatzis I, Konstantinidis S, et al. The anatomical relationship of inferior thyroid artery and recurrent laryngeal nerve: a review of the literature and its clinical importance. J Clin Med Res 2020;12(10):640–6.
43. Testini M, Gurrado A, Bellantone R, et al. Recurrent laryngeal nerve palsy and substernal goiter. An Italian multicenter study. J Visc Surg 2014;151(3):183–9.
44. White ML, Doherty GM, Gauger PG. Evidence-based surgical management of substernal goiter. World J Surg 2008;32(7):1285–300.

45. Gómez-Ramírez J, Sitges-Serra A, Moreno-Llorente P, et al. Mortality after thyroid surgery, insignificant or still an issue? Langenbeck's Arch Surg 2015;400(4): 517–22.
46. Landreneau RJ, Nawarawong W, Boley TM, et al. Intrathoracic goiter: approaching the posterior mediastinal mass. Ann Thorac Surg 1991;52(1):134–5, discussion 135-136.

Recurrent Laryngeal Nerve Monitoring: Nuts and Bolts

Diana N. Kirke, MD, MPhil, FRACS[a],
Catherine F. Sinclair, MD, FRACS, FACS[b,c,d],*

KEYWORDS

- Recurrent laryngeal nerve • Intraoperative nerve monitoring
- Intermittent intraoperative nerve monitoring
- Continuous intraoperative nerve monitoring

KEY POINTS

- Intermittent intraoperative neuromonitoring (IONM) is useful for localizing laryngeal nerves, determining when staged surgery may be necessary and defining types of nerve injury.
- Continuous IONM may be able to prevent slowly evolving forms of nerve injury and determining when staged surgery may be necessary.
- Continuous and intermittent monitoring are *complementary* techniques and optimally used together.
- Recent studies show a benefit of IONM in prevention of laryngeal nerve injury. The standardization of methodology and outcomes reporting for IONM will enhance reproducibility of future IONM clinical trials.

INTRODUCTION

Intraoperative neuromonitoring (IONM) of the laryngeal nerves has become an important tool for neck endocrine surgery. It is particularly important for thyroid surgery where commonly quoted rates of recurrent laryngeal nerve (RLN) injury are 1% to 5% and rates of external superior laryngeal nerve (EBSLN) injury are even higher. Although IONM use has increased significantly over the past decade, there remains variability in its utilization, largely due to past studies which presented data demonstrating no benefit of IONM over nerve visualization alone.[1] However, with standardization in IONM methodology and improved understanding of IONM principles, more recent trials have demonstrated benefits.[1-4]

---

[a] Department of Otolaryngology – Head & Neck Surgery, Icahn School of Medicine at Mount Sinai, One Gustave L Levy Place, Box 1189, Annenberg 10-40, New York, NY 10029, USA; [b] Department of Surgery, Monash University, Melbourne, Victoria, Australia; [c] Department of Otolaryngology – Head & Neck Surgery, Icahn School of Medicine at Mount Sinai, New York, NY, USA; [d] Melbourne Thyroid Surgery, 159 Wattletree Road, Malvern, Victoria 3144, Australia
* Corresponding author: Melbourne Thyroid Surgery, 159 Wattletree Road, Malvern, Melbourne, Victoria 3144, Australia.
E-mail address: Catherine@melbournethyroidsurgery.com.au

Otolaryngol Clin N Am 57 (2024) 53–61
https://doi.org/10.1016/j.otc.2023.08.002
0030-6665/24/© 2023 Elsevier Inc. All rights reserved.

With regard to IONM standardization, in 2011, the International Neural Monitoring Study Group (INMSG)[5] suggested the following sequence (**Box 1**) is followed to ensure consistency of results.

Such standardization has increased the use of IONM worldwide, and in a recent survey conducted across several global surgical societies, 83% of surgeons reported the use of IONM, with 18.1% of these reporting selective use.[6] Of note, 70.4% of North American surgeons used IONM consistently as opposed to 27.4% of surgeons in other parts of the world.[6] Despite these high rates of IONM use in North America, a recent survey of North American residents demonstrated a lack of didactic teaching and general understanding of IONM principles, indicating that improved education at more junior levels is necessary.[7]

In this article, the authors review the different forms of IONM, present the current evidence behind its use in neck endocrine procedures, and discuss recent advances in IONM and the importance of consistent outcomes reporting.

INTERMITTENT INTRAOPERATIVE NERVE MONITORING
Technique of Intermittent Intraoperative Nerve Monitoring

Intermittent RLN monitoring has been in robust clinical use for at least 2 decades. It is a surgeon-driven technique, performed with either a handheld neuroprobe (monopolar or bipolar) or dissector with connected stimulator that provides direct stimulation of the nerve. This stimulation elicits compound muscle action potentials (CMAPs) in the laryngeal muscles which are recorded on the endotracheal tube (ETT) surface electrodes.[2,4] Intermittent IONM (IIONM) is able to map out the course of the RLN before it being visualized and as such, can aid dissection by ensuring nonneural tissue only is divided. In the case of bilateral thyroid surgery, it can help prevent bilateral vocal fold (VF) injury by determining when staged surgery is appropriate in a loss of signal (LOS) event.[2] For IIONM to reliably serve these functions, it is important that the aforementioned L1/V1/R1/R2/V2 sequence is followed by the surgeon.

The general setup for IIONM has been extensively described in the literature. A brief summary follows. The type of general anesthesia is an important consideration in IONM of all forms and avoidance of long-acting paralytic agents by the anesthetic team is essential. Short-term neuromuscular blockade can be used at induction and the most widely used agent is succinylcholine which has a short half-life and does not interfere with eventual thyroid dissection and nerve localization. After intubation, the patient is positioned and the position of the ETT rechecked to ensure the electrodes are correctly placed within the larynx. During the surgical procedure, the current of the stimulation probe is most commonly set at 2 mA for mapping and vagus

---

Box 1
International neural monitoring study group recommendations

L1: Evaluation of preoperative vocal fold (VF) function on laryngoscopy

V1: Verification of vagal nerve (VN) functional integrity before dissection

R1: Verification of RLN functional integrity before dissection

R2: Verification of RLN functional integrity after dissection

V2: Verification of VN functional integrity after dissection

L2: Evaluation of postoperative VF function on laryngoscopy

nerve stimulation and 1 mA for direct RLN stimulation. Event threshold is generally set at 100 μV.[8] Stimulators that connect directly to a dissecting instrument have been recently developed and may improve surgical efficiency by eliminating the need to halt dissection while stimulating the nerve. In a study comparing handheld neuroprobes to dissector mounted stimulators, EMG amplitudes were comparable but speed of initial RLN identification was improved in the dissector group.[9]

Benefits

Overall, there are several benefits to using IIONM. These are summarized in **Box 2**.[4]

Despite these intuitive benefits, data demonstrating the impact of IIONM on reducing transient and permanent RLN injury have been conflicting. In a recent Cochrane review, there was no evidence of IIONM benefit in preventing permanent or transient RLN injury when compared with direct nerve visualization alone.[10] In a subsequent but larger randomized controlled trial (RCT) analysis, there was a trend toward significance for the use of IONM in preservation of overall RLN integrity but equivalence in the rates of transient and permanent RLN injury.[8] Possible reasons for the discrepancy in results between studies will be discussed in the final outcomes section of this article.

Limitations

In addition to the conjecture regarding its absolute benefit compared with visual identification alone, further limitations of IIONM include (**Box 3**) (1) the nerve is vulnerable to injury between the surgeon-driven stimulations (the so-called "limited in time" consideration)[11] which limits the ability of IIONM to actually "prevent" nerve injury; (2) the potential to miss a proximal RLN injury (the so-called "limited in space" consideration); and (3) potentially higher rates of transient VF paralysis and paresis compared with continuous IONM.[4,5]

These shortcomings of IIONM have led to the further refinement and evolution of IONM into its continuous forms as described below.

CONTINUOUS INTRAOPERATIVE NERVE MONITORING

During continuous IONM (CIONM) of the laryngeal nerves, electromyographic (EMG) signals are continuously generated from the VFs to provide real-time feedback about nerve functional integrity. Compared with IIONM, which relies on surgeon-driven nerve stimulation at discrete time points during surgery as discussed previously, CIONM information is obtained throughout a case such that there are no "gaps" or "windows" in the information provided. This allows the surgeon to know exactly how the nerve is behaving at any point in the surgery without having to stimulate it directly with a handheld or instrument-mounted neuroprobe.

Box 2
Benefits of intermittent intraoperative nerve monitoring

1. RLN localization

2. EBSLN localization

3. Distinguising whether a loss of signal has occurred and determining the type of loss of signal

4. Determining whether staged surgery is needed in a unilateral loss-of-signal event during planned bilateral central neck surgery

> **Box 3**
> **Limitations of intermittent intraoperative nerve monitoring**
>
> 1. Nerve is vulnerable in between stimulations, "limited in time"
> 2. May miss proximal injury, "limited in space"
> 3. Higher rates of transient nerve injury compared with CIONM

Techniques of Continuous Intraoperative Nerve Monitoring

Several techniques of CIONM have been trialed to date, with the two main approaches differing in both their site of stimulation and laryngeal EMG responses obtained. The first, and most well-publicized, method of CIONM uses one of several different types of vagus nerve electrodes to exert repetitive stimulation directly on the vagus nerve. Stimulation of the vagus nerve activates the vagus/RLN loop which results in VF adduction. Like IIONM, the EMG VF adduction response obtained during vagal electrode CIONM is a CMAP. Warning criteria and thresholds are similar to those described above for IIONM, with a 50% EMG amplitude decline combined with an increase in latency being most predictive of impending nerve injury. A recent comparative study of vagal CIONM versus IIONM during neck endocrine procedures was performed over a 10-year period. This study included 6029 patients with 5208 nerves at risk (NAR) monitored with CIONM, and 5024 NAR with IIONM. Vagal CIONM resulted in a 1.7-fold lower early VFP rates and 30-fold lower permanent VFP rates (0.02 vs 0.6%, respectively).[5] Similarly, a recent systematic review and meta-analysis on 23 papers showed a transient temporary RLN paralysis rate of 2.26% (95% CI: 1.6–2.9, $I^2 = 37$) and permanent RLN palsy rate of 0.05% (95% CI: 0.08–0.2, $I^2 = 0$). The study concluded that C-IONM is a safe and effective means by which RLN paralyses in thyroid surgery can be reduced.[12]

The main criticism of vagal CIONM is that placement of the vagus nerve electrode requires dissection into the carotid sheath, an area of the neck that is not usually dissected in routine thyroid surgery. The position of the vagus nerve in the carotid sheath is subject to interindividual variability and, particularly when the nerve runs posteriorly, isolating it to apply the electrode can be challenging and potentially dangerous, particularly through a small neck incision. There have been case reports of vagus nerve injury and decreased nerve potentials resulting from electrode placement and this has limited its widespread use in the thyroid community despite the potential advantages in reducing nerve injury rates.[13,14] In addition, once the electrode is placed around the vagus nerve, it can become dislodged by inadvertent traction on its connecting wire (particularly pertinent when operating through a small neck incision) which adds an extra "moving part" to the troubleshooting algorithm in the case of a LOS.

The other method of CIONM that is gradually gaining in popularity uses the laryngeal adductor reflex (LAR) to elicit VF adduction. The LAR is a primitive brainstem reflex that prevents aspiration of foreign objects into the tracheobronchial tree by initiating VF adduction. In contrast to IIONM and CIONM using vagus nerve electrodes, the EMG response obtained with LAR-CIONM is a reflex response that is distinct and separate from a CMAP (**Fig. 1**). This reflex response consists of two main EMG components: termed R1 and R2 as per neurophysiology standards for reflex reporting (see **Fig. 1**). Of note, it is essential to not confuse the LAR R1/R2 terminology with the R1/R2 terminology used by the INMSG as already described above, to describe surgical opening and closing RLN CMAP potentials. The LAR is elicited by supraglottic stimulation using ETT electrodes. Afferent information travels via the *internal* superior

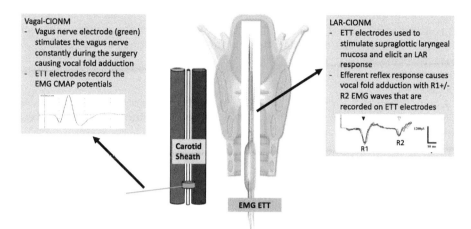

Fig. 1. Vagal continuous IONM versus laryngeal adductor reflex IONM (LAR-CIONM). ETT, endotracheal tube; EMG, electromyographic; CMAP, compound muscle action potential; LAR, laryngeal adductor reflex.

laryngeal nerve to the vagus nerve and brainstem nuclei. The efferent pathway involves bilateral vagus nerves and RLNs to the VFs, resulting in bilateral VF adduction. A recent case-historical control study comparing LAR-CIONM to IIONM reported an increased rate of postoperative transient VF paralysis and paresis in the I-IONM group.[4]

Advantages of LAR-CIONM compared with vagal CIONM include the absence of additional electrodes, avoidance of additional neck dissection, and ability to take baseline readings before skin incision. In addition, the ability to record bilateral VF EMG signals provides a potential troubleshooting mechanism for checking for ETT displacement and rotation. The main disadvantage of this technique at the current time is the lack of appropriately designed EMG ETTs for reliable reflex generation and the need to have a neurophysiologist in the room to perform the monitoring during surgery. These limitations will be overcome in the future as this technique is refined and further developed into single surgeon format.

Benefits

The benefits of CIONM (over intermittent forms of monitoring) relate to the continuous nature of the EMG information available to the surgeon at any point in time. If adverse changes in nerve potentials occur, a surgeon using CIONM will be able to potentially alter their surgical strategy *at the time the changes are occurring*. This alteration in strategy may involve releasing tension on retracted tissue, changing the angle/strength of retraction, ceasing dissection and resting the nerve, and/or irrigating the surgical field. The surgeon can then watch and wait for nerve recovery before continuing the procedure. Over time, ongoing recognition of the EMG amplitude decline that regularly occurs with certain surgical maneuvers can change surgical strategy, subsequently altering how the surgery is performed to minimize frequency and duration of EMG declines. CIONM can also provide information on the time course of any given nerve injury and, as for IIONM, can help determine when to stage a total thyroidectomy in the case of unilateral LOS.

Limitations

Unlike IIONM, CIONM cannot help localize a nerve, identify aberrant branching patterns, nor distinguish between Type 1 (segmental) and Type 1 (global) LOS injuries.

It also cannot prevent injuries due to sudden mechanisms such as transection and ligation as the time course of injury will be too rapid to enable surgeon driven alteration in surgical strategy. Also, CIONM techniques are also only as good as the surgeon using them—if the surgeon chooses not to respond or does not understand the information provided, the ability of CIONM to prevent evolving nerve injury will be compromised.

A comparison of the strengths of IIONM versus CIONM is presented in **Fig. 2**. As noted in the figure, these techniques are *complementary* to each other and are best used together.

ADVANCES IN INTRAOPERATIVE NERVE MONITORING

There have been several recent studies looking at the feasibility of transcutaneous or needle stimulation and recording of EMG potentials during thyroid surgery and ablative procedures.[15–17] These studies have investigated the optimum point of placement of electrodes and quality of the EMG signals obtained. In general, EMG amplitudes obtained transcutaneously are lower in amplitude than those obtained from the EMG ETT, however, seem clinically usable, particularly when placed over the lateral thyroid lamina. Transcartilaginous and transcricothyroid membrane electrode potentials are more comparable to those obtained on the EMG ETT. The main issues with transcutaneous and needle methodologies again relate to electrode displacement during surgery and, for needle methodologies, possibility of damage to laryngeal structures during needle insertion. For remote access thyroidectomy approaches, one recent trial evaluated percutaneous continuous vagus nerve stimulation in 325 nerves-at-risk during robotic thyroidectomy via the bilateral axillo-breast approach. They concluded that this was a feasible approach that avoided additional trocar space and repeated instrument changes.[18]

CONTROVERSIES IN INTRAOPERATIVE NERVE MONITORING: WHAT OUTCOMES SHOULD WE MEASURE?

There has been controversy over past decades as to whether IONM (particularly IIONM) is better than visual nerve identification alone. Multiple studies have shown conflicting results, with some citing no difference between subgroups and some

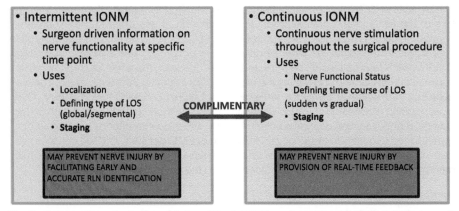

Fig. 2. Comparative strengths of intermittent IONM and continuous IONM. LOS, loss of signal.

Table 1
Appropriate outcomes to measure for intermittent and continuous forms of intraoperative neuromonitoring

Type of IONM	Appropriate Outcomes to Measure
IIONM	• Pre- and post-dissection vagal/RLN trace amplitudes and latencies (V1R1R2V2) • Classification of any LOS into segmental vs global • Correlation between closing signal reductions and postoperative laryngeal function • Rates of bilateral vocal fold palsy • The utility of IIONM in RLN localization and identification of anatomic variants • The utility of IIONM to localize the EBSLN and verify the functional integrity pre- and post-superior pole dissection
CIONM	• Rates of temporary and permanent vocal fold paralysis • Rates of unrecoverable vs recoverable intraoperative LOS and postoperative vocal fold paralysis (VFP) • Time course of injury for any given LOS • Rates of bilateral vocal fold injury

noting significant benefits. The primary outcome measure in all these studies has been rates of postoperative VF paralysis. However, as discussed above, the ability of intermittent forms of IONM to *prevent* nerve injury is limited by their intermittent nature which does not allow for complete real-time knowledge of nerve functional integrity. As such, although IIONM may be helpful in preventing nerve injury by virtue of its localization abilities in certain situations such as revision surgery and anatomically aberrant nerves, there are other benefits that are important to note when reporting outcomes for IIONM. Defining the correct outcomes to measure when evaluating IONM techniques was the subject of a recent consensus statement from the American Head and Neck Society.[19] The conclusions of this statement are tabulated in **Table 1**.

In accord with these recommendations, a recent systematic review and meta-analysis of seven studies with 19,047 patients evaluated the diagnostic accuracy of IIONM and CIONM in *predicting* VFP postoperatively.[20] Using this outcome measure, both forms of IONM displayed excellent diagnostic accuracy, although diagnostic accuracy was highest in the CIONM group. Interestingly, on subgroup analysis, articles published after 2011 had notably higher diagnostic accuracy than earlier publications (<2010), likely reflecting the successful efforts to standardize of IONM methodology over the past decade.

SUMMARY

Methodologies and techniques of IONM are continuing to evolve. Recent publications suggest that there is a benefit to using IONM over no monitoring at all with respect to postoperative nerve injury rates, although continuous forms of IONM are likely better able to prevent nerve injuries than intermittent forms. The benefits of IONM can be best demonstrated when its effect on outcomes in addition to VF paralysis are considered.

CLINICS CARE POINTS

- Intermittent techniques of neuromonitoring are useful for localizing nerves and determining when staged surgery may be required in the case of a loss of signal. However,

- the ability of intermittent monitoring to *prevent* nerve injury is limited by virtue of its intermittent, surgeon-driven nature.
- Recent large meta-analyses and clinical trials have showed improved nerve palsy rates with continuous forms of nerve monitoring over intermittent forms.
- The temporal course of any nerve injury is an important consideration when determining whether neuromonitoring can play a preventative role—slowly evolving injuries are best able to be prevented, whereas sudden injuries (such as transection) will not be prevented by any form of monitoring
- Intraoperative neuromonitoring of any form is only as good as the surgeon using it; surgeons should ensure that they are comfortable with troubleshooting algorithms and methodologies and that they are prepared to identify and act on any information provided to them by the nerve monitoring equipment.

CONFLICTS OF INTEREST

None.

FINANCIAL DISCLOSURES

C. Sinclair Inventor is named on a patent held by Mount Sinai Innovation Partners, filed on 12/23/2016, entitled "Improved Method and System for Assessing Laryngeal and Vagus Nerve Integrity in Patients Under General Anesthesia. No funds have been received from this patent.

REFERENCES

1. Grishaeva P, Kussmann J, Burgstaller T, et al. Recurrent laryngeal nerve paresis in benign thyroid surgery with and without intraoperative nerve monitoring. Minerva Surg 2022;77(6):558–63.
2. Randolph GW, Dralle H. International Neuromonitoring Study Group Electrophysiologic recurrent laryngeal nerve monitoring during thyroid and parathyroid surgery: international standards guideline statement. Laryngoscope 2011; 121(Suppl 1):S1–16.
3. Sinclair CF, Téllez MJ, Ulkatan S. Continuous Laryngeal Adductor Reflex Versus Intermittent Nerve Monitoring in Neck Endocrine Surgery. Laryngoscope 2021; 131(1):230–6.
4. Schneider R, Machens A, Sekulla C, et al. Superiority of continuous over intermittent intraoperative nerve monitoring in preventing vocal cord palsy. Br J Surg 2021;108(5):566–73.
5. Davey MG, Cleere EF, Lowery AJ, et al. Intraoperative recurrent laryngeal nerve monitoring versus visualisation alone - A systematic review and meta-analysis of randomized controlled trials. Am J Surg 2022;224(3):836–41. Epub 2022 Apr 9. PMID: 35422329.
6. Feng AL, Puram SV, Singer MC, et al. Increased prevalence of neural monitoring during thyroidectomy: Global surgical survey. Laryngoscope 2020;130(4): 1097–104. Epub 2019 Jul 30. PMID: 31361342.
7. Wong A, Ahsanuddin S, Teng M, et al. US residents experiences with intraoperative nerve monitoring in thyroid and parathyroid surgery. Head Neck 2023;45(8): 2009–16. Epub 2023 Jun 9. PMID: 37293876.
8. Bartsch DK, Dotzenrath C, Vorländer C, et al. The StuDoQ/Thyroid Study Group TSS. Current Practice of Surgery for Benign Goitre-An Analysis of the Prospective

DGAV StuDoQ|Thyroid Registry. J Clin Med 2019;8(4):477. PMID: 30965665; PMCID: PMC6517925.

9. Karaisli S, Gucek Haciyanli S, Haciyanli M. Comparison of stimulating dissector and intermittent stimulating probe for the identification of recurrent laryngeal nerve in reoperative setting. Eur Arch Oto-Rhino-Laryngol 2022;279:443–7.

10. Cirocchi R, Arezzo A, D'Andrea V, et al. Intraoperative Neuromonitoring Versus Visual Nerve Identification for Prevention of Recurrent Laryngeal Nerve Injury in Adults Undergoing Thyroid Surgery. Cochrane Database Syst Rev 2019;1: CD012483. https://doi.org/10.1002/14651858.CD012483.

11. Schneider R, Machens A, Randolph GW, et al. Opportunities and challenges of intermittent and continuous intraoperative neural monitoring in thyroid surgery. Gland Surg 2017;6(5):537–45.

12. Ku D, Hui M, Cheung P, et al. Meta-analysis on continuous nerve monitoring in thyroidectomies. Head Neck 2021;43(12):3966–78. Epub 2021 Aug 3. PMID: 34342380.

13. Mathieson T, Jimaja W, Triponez F, et al. Safety of continuous intraoperative vagus nerve neuromonitoring during thyroid surgery. BJS Open 2023;7(3). zrad039.

14. Terris DJ, Chaung K, Duke WS. Continuous Vagal Nerve Monitoring is Dangerous and Should not Routinely be Done During Thyroid Surgery. World J Surg 2015; 39(10):2471–6.

15. Shin SC, Sung ES, Kwon HK, et al. Investigation of attachment location of adhesive skin electrodes for intraoperative neuromonitoring in thyroid surgery: Preclinical and clinical studies. Surgery 2022;171(2):377–83. Epub 2021 Sep 22. PMID: 34563352.

16. McManus C, Kuo JH. Intraoperative Neuromonitoring: Evaluating the Role of Continuous IONM and IONM Techniques for Emerging Surgical and Percutaneous Procedures. Front Endocrinol 2022;13:808107.

17. Xu C, Wang X, Liu J, et al. The Feasibility Study of Intraoperative RLN Monitoring Using Cricothyroid Membrane-Inserted Needle Electrodes During Thyroid Surgery. Otolaryngol Head Neck Surg 2023. https://doi.org/10.1002/ohn.338.

18. Zhang D, Wang C, Wang T, et al. Clinical experience of use of percutaneous continuous nerve monitoring in robotic bilateral axillo-breast thyroid surgery. Front Endocrinol 2022;12:817026.

19. Sinclair CF, Buczek E, Cottril E, et al. Clarifying optimal outcome measures in intermittent and continuous laryngeal neuromonitoring. Head Neck 2022;44(2): 460–71.

20. Kim DH, Kim SW, Hwang SH. Intraoperative Neural Monitoring for Early Vocal Cord Function Assessment After Thyroid Surgery: A Systematic Review and Meta-Analysis. World J Surg 2021;45(11):3320–7.

Avoiding Complications of Thyroidectomy
Preservation of Parathyroid Glands

Elizabeth E. Cottrill, MD

KEYWORDS

- Parathyroid preservation • Hypoparathyroidism • Autofluorescence

KEY POINTS

- Knowledge of embryology and anatomy is foundational to parathyroid preservation without devascularization.
- Anticipatory dissection immediately on the thyroid capsule medial and ventral to the parathyroids allows for their identification and preservation of their blood supply.
- When avulsion or devascularization occurs, autotransplantation should be undertaken.
- Technologies harnessing autofluorescent properties of parathyroid tissue can aid in identification of parathyroid glands intraoperatively, but do not assess for viable tissue.
- Indocyanine green angiography can assess the adequacy of vascular supply to parathyroids intraoperatively.

INTRODUCTION

Preservation of the parathyroid glands during thyroid surgery and/or central neck dissection is a critical aspect of the procedure that must be performed deliberately to minimize the risk of postoperative hypoparathyroidism (hypoPT), a common and potentially life-threatening complication. HypoPT can occur due to removal or devascularization of the parathyroid glands during surgery. Herein, we discuss techniques that can be used to preserve the parathyroid glands during surgery, factors that influence the success of these techniques, and new technologies that may be used to aid in recognition and potentially preservation of parathyroid tissue.

Background

hypoPT is one of the most common complications of total thyroidectomy, completion thyroidectomy, and surgeries involving bilateral central compartment neck dissection.[1–5] The incidence of postsurgical hypoPT is difficult to know definitively because

Department of Otolaryngology Head and Neck Surgery, Thomas Jefferson University Hospital, 925 Chestnut Street. 6th Floor, Philadelphia, PA 19107, USA
E-mail address: Elizabeth.cottrill@jefferson.edu

Otolaryngol Clin N Am 57 (2024) 63–74
https://doi.org/10.1016/j.otc.2023.07.009
0030-6665/24/© 2023 Elsevier Inc. All rights reserved.

of the variety and extent of the procedures performed, various postoperative supplementation protocols, and varying clinical and biochemical criteria used to evaluate or define it.[1,6–8] A 2018 position statement from the American Thyroid Association defined temporary hypoPT, as an intact parathyroid hormone (PTH) level less than the lower limit of the laboratory standard (usually 12 pg/mL) concurrent with resultant hypocalcemia for less than 6 months after surgery and defined permanent hypoPT as this condition lasting beyond 6 months.[1] A 2014 systematic review and meta-analysis of 116 studies estimated the median incidence of temporary hypoPT ranges from 19% to 38% and permanent hypoPT 0% to 3%.[8] Risk factors for postoperative hypoPT have been evaluated by many authors and are summarized in **Box 1**.[8–10]

Embryology and Anatomy

The first step in the recognition and preservation of parathyroid glands during central neck surgery is development of a solid foundational knowledge of parathyroid embryology and anatomy. The development of the parathyroid glands starts during the fourth week of embryonic development. They arise from the third and fourth pharyngeal pouches, which also give rise to other structures. The third pharyngeal pouch gives rise to the inferior parathyroid glands as well as the thymus, whereas the fourth pharyngeal pouch gives rise to the superior parathyroid glands, thus the parathyroid pairs are occasionally referenced as PIII and PIV, respectively. The migration of the parathyroid cells to their final location occurs during the seventh week of embryonic development.[11,12]

The parathyroid glands are highly vascularized. Although classic teaching is that parathyroids are dominantly supplied by the inferior thyroid artery, Halstead and Evans[13] and more recently Nobori and colleagues have described superior thyroid artery contributions to parathyroid vascularity[14] (**Fig. 1**). Parathyroid glands are innervated by sympathetic and parasympathetic fibers.[15]

Owing to embryologic migration, the parathyroid glands may have variable final anatomic location (**Table 1**). The superior parathyroid glands (PIV) are most often located at the level of the cricoid cartilage or the lower border of the thyroid cartilage, whereas the inferior parathyroid glands (PIII) are often located at the level of the junction between the inferior and middle thirds of the thyroid gland.[11] Because of the longer migration tract of the PIII glands, from the level of the mandible to the pericardium, their normal location includes a wider area and they are also more likely to be ectopic. Undescended PIIIs can be located high in the neck above the thyroid along the carotid sheath often along with a remnant of thymic tissue.[16,19,26] Contrary to their

---

Box 1
Risk factors for permanent hypoparathyroidism following central neck operations:

Bilateral thyroid procedures (total thyroidectomy or completion)

Central Neck Dissection

Autoimmune thyroiditis (Graves' disease, chronic lymphocytic thyroiditis)

Substernal goiter

Low-volume thyroid surgeon

Prior gastric bypass or malabsorptive state

Simultaneous thyroidectomy and parathyroidectomy

Prior central neck surgery/revision central neck surgery

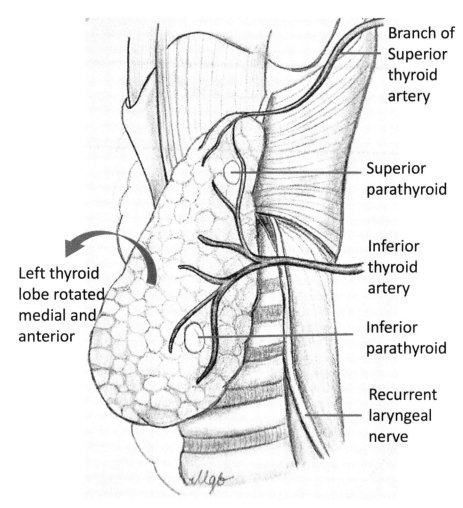

Fig. 1. Parathyroid vascularization with branches from both inferior and superior thyroid arteries depicted. Preservation of viable parathyroid glands requires maintaining an adequate blood supply through the distal branches which supply them. (Image courtesy: Isabella Boon.)

naming, the superior parathyroid glands are not always found cephalad to the inferior glands, but the pairs do maintain a consistent anatomic relationship to each other as they relate to the course of the recurrent laryngeal nerve: the superior glands (PIV) being located *posterior or dorsal* to the trajectory of the nerve and the inferior glands (PIII) being *anteriorly or ventrally* located.

The parathyroid glands may be located within the fibrofatty tissue in the thyroid bed, adherent to the thyroid capsule, *within* the thyroid capsule, or rarely intrathyroidal. A true intrathyroidal parathyroid, fully embedded in thyroid parenchyma, is extremely rare and should be distinguished from a parathyroid which is located just beneath the thyroid capsule (subcapsular) and is less rare. The historically reported incidence of a true intrathyroidal parathyroid is between 0.5% and 4%.[16,18,24,27] More recent studies have reported the prevalence of intrathyroidal parathyroids to be more common on the right side and within the inferior portion of the thyroid lobe, and their

Table 1
Parathyroid gland location

Superior Parathyroid (PIII)	References	Inferior Parathyroid (PIV)	References
80% posterior aspect of thyroid lobe, 1 cm cephalad to the intersection of the inferior thyroid artery and the recurrent laryngeal nerve, close to the cricothyroid joint	Refs[16–18]	42%–61% along the anterior, lateral, or posterior aspect of the inferior thyroid pole	Refs[18, 19]
15% posterolateral surface of the superior thyroid pole	Refs[16,18,20,21]	25% thyrothymic ligament or within the cervical thymus	Ref[18]
3%–4% retropharyngeal or retroesophageal	Refs[16,18]	5% anterior mediastinum or intrathoracic	Refs[16, 18,22]
<1% cephalad to the superior pole of the thyroid: adjacent to carotid, pyriform sinus, and so forth	Refs[18,23,24]	2% cephalad ectopic position above superior pole (easily confused with PIVs) <4% intrathyroidal (most common right inferior pole)	Refs[16, 18,19,22,25]

frequency is reportedly higher in cases of hyperfunctioning parathyroid glands.[28,29] Although there is considerable variability in the final location of the parathyroid glands, there is often mirror symmetry from right to left with symmetry of the PIV seen in approximately 80% of cases and of the PIII in approximately 70% of cases. The most common asymmetry identified is when one PIII is located within the thymus. The awareness of parathyroid symmetry may facilitate parathyroid gland identification during surgical neck exploration.

Supernumerary and subnumerary parathyroid glands are also possible. Autopsy series have reported less than four glands in up to 6% of the population,[4,21] potentially an overestimate given the frequency of ectopic glands which may not have been identified. More than four glands have been reported in 5% to 13% of autopsies with up to 11 distinct parathyroids being reported in a single individual.[18,30,31] In patients with renally induced hyperparathyroidism (HPT) reports are higher. A study of 300 renal-HPT patients reported 30% of patients having more than four parathyroids identified at the time of initial surgery with 80% of these being located in the cervical thymus.[30] These supernumerary parathyroid glands develop from accessory parathyroid fragments arising from the pharyngobranchial duct when the pharyngeal pouches separate from the pharynx.[26] Microscopic ectopic rests are also somewhat common. These are derived from embryologic parathyroid debris and weigh less than 5 mg as compared with true supernumerary parathyroids which weigh 24 g on average.[18] A 1992 study of surgical patients without renal HPT reported finding microscopic embryonic parathyroid rests in less than 30% of patients.[32] In the case of HPT, the presence of continuous growth stimulation may stimulate microscopic rests to grow and thus reaches a size comparable to true supernumerary glands.[18,31]

Intraoperative Technique

The perspicacious surgeon builds on a solid foundational anatomic and embryologic knowledge with the practice of meticulous surgical technique. Avoiding damage to the parathyroid glands first requires that a surgeon can recognize parathyroid tissue to avoid avulsing it from its blood supply. Unfortunately, parathyroid glands can appear deceptively similar to fibroadipose tissue, lymph nodes, and even thyroid tissue due to their small size, coloration, and the classic presence of a fat-cap. Therefore, using anatomic and embryologic foundational knowledge as a basic map, one is able to identify landmarks and use a "proactive anticipatory visual approach,"[1] in the words of Orloff and colleagues to identify parathyroid tissue.

The technique of gentle capsular dissection, immediately on the surface of the thyroid, reflecting the perithyroidal fatty tissues serially as one works from medial to lateral and from ventral to dorsal along the capsule of the thyroid allows for identification and preservation of the parathyroid blood supply in the majority of cases. There is evidence that utilization of loupe magnification (2.5x) significantly reduces the rate of inadvertent parathyroidectomy (3.8% vs 7.8%) and both postoperative clinical and biochemical hypocalcemia.[33] It should be emphasized that surgical technique requires dissection immediately on the surface of the thyroid gland medial or anterior to the parathyroids and therefore distal to their fine network of blood supply (see **Fig. 1**). One should anticipate the possible arterial contribution of the superior thyroid artery via a small branch to the superior parathyroid as well as anastomotic branches and care should be taken to preserve these contributions during dissection of the superior thyroid pole. Once identified, the parathyroids are carefully freed from their medial attachments and reflected off the thyroid gland along with their laterally based vascular pedicle while ligating only the distal-most branches of the inferior thyroid artery at the level of the thyroid capsule.[34] Vessels spanning the medial border of the parathyroid and the adjacent lateral thyroid capsule are generally believed to be insufficient to vascularize the parathyroid gland and it has been suggested that distal arterial segments may be supplied by anastomotic vessels from the trachea and esophagus.[34,35] Nevertheless, a classic 1982 study by Delattre and colleagues of 100 cadaveric dissections of the neck injected with latex to study the vascular supply of the parathyroids reported that standard capsular dissection would likely have been insufficient to maintain vascular supply to all four parathyroids in 5.5% of specimens.[36]

The use of energy devices for vessel sealing during thyroidectomy is another relevant surgical technical factor. These energy devices generate a zone of collateral thermal spread within the tissues and necessitate an optimal 3 to 5 mm distance of separation between the instrument and the parathyroid gland to avoid thermal injury to adjacent tissues.[37,38] After removal of the specimen, it should be critically inspected for evidence of adherent parathyroid tissue before handing off the specimen for pathology. Any avulsed parathyroid tissue should be immediately placed in cold saline for preservation and consideration of confirmation of parathyroid tissue via frozen section or other modality (see next section discussing technologies) before preparing it for auto transplantation.

Visual inspection of the parathyroid glands in vivo after extirpation of the thyroid or central lymph node packet should be undertaken critically to assess for devascularization or venous congestion. Venous disruption can often be perceived visually by classic darkening and implies the high potential for dysfunction of that gland. A parathyroid which is found to have apparent blood supply, but dark blue–purple discoloration may have vascular congestion which can often be alleviated by sharp scoring of the parathyroid gland capsule resulting in normalization of color. Care should be taken not to disrupt the blood supply in performing this maneuver and a fresh blade or sharp scissor which has not been in contact with cancerous tissue should be used. In turn, the blade or scissor used for scoring should then be either cleaned or retired for the duration of the case to avoid the risk of inadvertent parathyroid auto transplantation. Arterial ischemia of the parathyroid may be subtle or without any perceptible color change. indocyanine green (ICG) angiography, discussed later, is a newer technology which may be used to evaluate parathyroid tissue more clearly for appropriate vascular function. Although frank avulsion from blood supply is a clear indication for autotransplantation, some studies suggest that discolored parathyroids have only transiently impaired function,[39,40] recommending autotransplantation only if the evidence of arterial insufficiency is clearly seen or confirmed by angiography.

Preservation of intrathyroidal parathyroids as well as those located within the thyroid capsule is incredibly difficult and, especially in the case of the former, would likely require high suspicion on preoperative ultrasonographic imaging. If a subcapsular parathyroid is identified after removal of the thyroid gland, consideration of the proximity of the parathyroid to a potentially cancerous thyroid nodule should be made before incising the thyroid capsule to remove the parathyroid for reimplantation. Generally, a small intraoperative biopsy should be undertaken to confirm parathyroid tissue before morselization and reimplantation.

Although preservation of all parathyroid glands during total thyroidectomy with or without central neck dissection is a critically important operative goal, this objective is not always attainable due to potential variations in location or blood supply of the glands or due to the extent of thyroid disease such as in the case of thyroid cancer with a high burden of central neck metastases. During central neck dissection, superior parathyroid glands are at lower risk of devascularization or inadvertent removal than the inferior glands, owing to the bulk of nodal metastases being in the more caudal paratracheal and pre-tracheal areas. If central neck dissection is to be undertaken, this author recommends using a 5 to 0 Prolene to mark the parathyroids opposite their vascular pedicle at the time of their initial identification to help identify them clearly during dissection of level VI. If autofluorescent technology (discussed later) is available, then this technology along with surgeon visualization to confirm parathyroid tissue can be used. If avulsed or devascularized parathyroid glands are not overtly involved with cancer, then morselization and autotransplantation in the sternocleidomastoid muscle should be undertaken. Consideration should be given to staged or less aggressive contralateral surgery if there is evidence of devascularization of both parathyroids on one side requiring autotransplantation.

Technological Advances: Autofluorescence and Parathyroid Angiography

New technology, aimed at improving identification of parathyroid glands intraoperatively, has arisen over the past 10 to 15 years. Researchers at Vanderbilt University discovered that when excited in the near-infrared (NIR) spectrum (785 nm), the resulting autofluorescence (AF) wavelength of parathyroid tissue (820–830 nm) was consistently greater than that of surrounding tissue types (thyroid, fat, and muscle).[41] Technologies which harness this natural phenomenon rely on the *difference* between emitted wavelengths of tissues in the central neck. The technologies use either a camera with visual comparison of exposed tissues by the surgeon in real time, or a disposable probe which measures the AF wavelength of the tissue being touched. NIR-AF technology is noninvasive and real time. It requires no drugs or injections, thus avoiding side-effects. The two kinds of NIR-AF systems which currently exist are detailed in **Table 2** and these include both a probe-based system (PTEye, Medtronic) and an optical-based system (Fluobeam, Fluoptics). Other commercially available optical systems exist and can also be used for parathyroid detection, although not FDA approved for this use specifically.[42]

Because the technology relies on the difference in AF wavelengths between tissues, it is important to realize several limitations.

- AF intensity may differ between patients.
- Diseased parathyroids (hyperplasia, adenomas) may have weaker AF than normal glands.
- Thyroid tissue can have abnormally high AF, especially in the case of thyroiditis
- False-positive signals have been reported from colloid nodules, brown fat, and metastatic lymph nodes.[43]
- The fluorophore intrinsic to parathyroid tissue is present in vivo and ex vivo and is resistant to heat, freezing, and formalin fixation,[44–46] therefore, these technologies do not assess viability or vascular supply of the tissue.

Table 2
Comparison of near-infrared autofluorescence systems available in the United States

Probe-Based Spectroscopy	Optical Camera-Based
• Surgeon holds a sterile probe • Background level is calibrated from five separate locations on the thyroid or trachea • System analyzes optical properties of the tissue being touched and gives a distinct numeric reading as well as audio/visual feedback • FDA-approved device (2018): PTEye (MedTronic)	• Surgeon looks at operative field with special camera within a sterile sheath • Surgeon visually searches for foci of high autofluorescence as compared with background • Imaging is limited to superficial layers of tissue • FDA-approved device (2018): Fluobeam (Fluoptics)

Despite these limitations, many studies over the past 8 years have shown the high accuracy and clinical usefulness of this technology.[44,45,47–65] Most of these studies report that the identification of parathyroid glands is more accurate with AF-based systems than with the naked eye only and allow for identification of parathyroid glands which would otherwise have been missed. Several studies also report better postoperative outcomes regarding hypoPT when using NIR-AF modalities.[50,57,64,66,67]

As mentioned previously, visual detection of ischemic parathyroid glands is imperfect and given the persistence of AF properties in devascularized and even formalin fixed parathyroid tissue, viability of parathyroids cannot be confirmed with NIR-AF technologies. Angiography with the fluorescent dye ICG has therefore been developed to confirm perfusion of parathyroid glands in vivo. ICG is an albumin-bound, water-soluble fluorescent dye with a half-life of 2 to 3 minutes and is FDA-approved. It was initially used to evaluate liver function and currently is used for retinochoroidal angiography. It has a peak absorption at 800 nm and peak emission at 830 nm, in the NIR spectrum, and can penetrate tissues up to 1 cm in depth allowing excellent visualization of vascularity. Owing to its short half-life and a toxic dose of 5 mg/kg, it can theoretically be injected many times throughout a procedure. The technology necessary to perform intraoperative ICG angiography is often readily available as most modern institutions in the United States will be equipped with an ICG fluorescence endoscopic camera in their operating suites. Its limitations are inherent in the lack of standardization and subjective nature of the assessment with currently available devices lacking numerical evaluation. It is therefore difficult to concretely compare data between groups or assess differences between devices used.[68,69]

Several studies have reported that ICG angiography is superior to "naked eye" visualization alone in determining vascular supply to the parathyroid glands and the correlation between vascularization and parathyroid function postoperatively has a very high positive predictive value.[70–73] ICG angiography can be used to evaluate parathyroid vasculature after thyroidectomy or paratracheal dissection, but it can also be used to identify the parathyroid vessel before thyroid resection allowing the surgeon to spare vessels which would otherwise have been ligated. This method of vessel mapping is an area of ongoing research.[57,74,75] Some studies have suggested that if at least one parathyroid gland is well-vascularized, the patient may be managed without measuring calcium and PTH postoperatively.[70]

DISCLOSURE

E.E. Cottrill does not have any commercial or financial relationships or conflicts of interest to disclose.

REFERENCES

1. Orloff LA, Wiseman SM, Bernet VJ, et al. American Thyroid Association Statement on Postoperative Hypoparathyroidism: Diagnosis, Prevention, and Management in Adults. Thyroid 2018;28(7):830–41.
2. Ho TWT, Shaheen AA, Dixon E, et al. Utilization of thyroidectomy for benign disease in the United States: a 15-year population-based study. Am J Surg 2011; 201(5):570–4.
3. Hauch A, Al-Qurayshi Z, Randolph G, et al. Total Thyroidectomy is Associated with Increased Risk of Complications for Low- and High-Volume Surgeons. Ann Surg Oncol 2014;21(12):3844–52.
4. Brandi ML, Bilezikian JP, Shoback D, et al. Management of Hypoparathyroidism: Summary Statement and Guidelines. J Clin Endocrinol Metab 2016;101(6):2273–83.

5. Bollerslev J, Rejnmark L, Marcocci C, et al. European Society of Endocrinology Clinical Guideline: Treatment of chronic hypoparathyroidism in adults. Eur J Endocrinol 2015;173(2):G1–20.
6. Lorente-Poch L, Sancho JJ, Muñoz-Nova JL, et al. Defining the syndromes of parathyroid failure after total thyroidectomy. Gland Surg 2015;4(1):82–90.
7. Postoperative hypocalcemia—The difference a definition makes - Mehanna - 2010 - Head & Neck - Wiley Online Library. Available at: https://onlinelibrary.wiley.com/doi/abs/10.1002/hed.21175?casa_token=19DxdQsNXY8AAAAA:v-tlhAEzzbxOKKLX TkboW7r-IClqyWFH0G5AYbR HD2XVLj2wDigkqjo2Fqi2znc_57NUkzqW_aWlFc. Accessed June 4, 2023.
8. Edafe O, Antakia R, Laskar N, et al. Systematic review and meta-analysis of predictors of post-thyroidectomy hypocalcaemia. Br J Surg 2014;101(4):307–20.
9. Thomusch O, Machens A, Sekulla C, et al. Multivariate Analysis of Risk Factors for Postoperative Complications in Benign Goiter Surgery: Prospective Multicenter Study in Germany. World J Surg 2000;24(11):1335–41.
10. Chen Z, Zhao Q, Du J, et al. Risk factors for postoperative hypocalcaemia after thyroidectomy: A systematic review and meta-analysis. J Int Med Res 2021; 49(3). 300060521996911.
11. Randolph G. Surgery of the thyroid and parathyroid glands. 3rd edition. Philadelphia, PA: Elsevier; 2021.
12. Tortora GJ. Principles of anatomy & physiology. 14th edition. Danvers, MA: Wiley; 2014.
13. Halsted WS, Evans HMI. The Parathyroid Glandules. Their Blood Supply and their Preservation in Operation upon the Thyroid Gland. Ann Surg 1907;46(4):489–506.
14. Nobori M, Saiki S, Tanaka N, et al. Blood supply of the parathyroid gland from the superior thyroid artery. Surgery 1994;115(4):417–23.
15. Gray H, Standring S, Anhand N. In: *Gray's anatomy: the anatomical basis of clinical practice*. 42nd edition. Amsterdam: Elsevier; 2021.
16. Wang C. The anatomic basis of parathyroid surgery. Ann Surg 1976;183(3): 271–5.
17. Gilmour JR. The gross anatomy of the parathyroid glands. J Pathol Bacteriol 1938;46(1):133–49.
18. Akerström G, Malmaeus J, Bergström R. Surgical anatomy of human parathyroid glands. Surgery 1984;95(1):14–21.
19. Edis AJ, Purnell DC, van Heerden JA. The undescended "parathymus". An occasional cause of failed neck exploration for hyperparathyroidism. Ann Surg 1979; 190(1):64–8.
20. Thompson NW, Eckhauser FE, Harness JK. The anatomy of primary hyperparathyroidism. Surgery 1982;92(5):814–21.
21. Randolph GW, Grant CS, Kamani D. Principles in surgical management of primary hyperparathyroidism. Surg thyroid parathyr glands. 2nd edition. Philadelphia: Elsevier Saunders; 2013. p. 546–66.
22. Henry J. Surgical anatomy and embryology of the thyroid and parathyroid glands and recurrent and external laryngeal nerves. In: Clark OH, Duh QY, Kebebew E, editors. Textbook of endocrine surgery. Philadelphia, PA: Elsevier; 2005. p. 9–15.
23. Chan TJ, Libutti SK, McCart JA, et al. Persistent Primary Hyperparathyroidism Caused by Adenomas Identified in Pharyngeal or Adjacent Structures. World J Surg 2003;27(6):675–9.
24. Fukumoto A, Nonaka M, Kamio T, et al. A case of ectopic parathyroid gland hyperplasia in the pyriform sinus. Arch Otolaryngol Head Neck Surg 2002;128(1):71–4.

25. Peissig K, Condie BG, Manley NR. Embryology of the Parathyroid Glands. Endocrinol Metab Clin North Am 2018;47(4):733–42.
26. Pradhan R, Agarwal A, Lombardi CP, et al. Applied embryology of the thyroid and parathyroid glands. In: Surgery of the thyroid and parathyroid glands. Elsevier; 2021. p. 15–25.e4.
27. Wheeler MH, Williams ED, Wade JS. The hyperfunctioning intrathyroidal parathyroid gland: a potential pitfall in parathyroid surgery. World J Surg 1987;11(1): 110–4.
28. Ros S, Sitges-Serra A, Pereira JA, et al. [Intrathyroid parathyroid adenomas: right and lower]. Cir Esp 2008;84(4):196–200.
29. Proye C, Bizard JP, Carnaille B, et al. [Hyperparathyroidism and intrathyroid parathyroid gland. 43 cases]. Ann Chir 1994;48(6):501–6.
30. Pattou FN, Pellissier LC, Noël C, et al. Supernumerary Parathyroid Glands: Frequency and Surgical Significance in Treatment of Renal Hyperparathyroidism. World J Surg 2000;24(11):1330–4.
31. Aly A, Douglas M. Embryonic parathyroid rests occur commonly and have implications in the management of secondary hyperparathyroidism. ANZ J Surg 2003; 73(5):284–8.
32. Kraimps JL, Duh QY, Demeure M, et al. Hyperparathyroidism in multiple endocrine neoplasia syndrome. Surgery 1992;112(6):1080–8.
33. Pata G, Casella C, Mittempergher F, et al. Loupe magnification reduces postoperative hypocalcemia after total thyroidectomy. Am Surg 2010;76(12):1345–50.
34. Attie JN. Primary hyperparathyroidism. Curr Ther Endocrinol Metab 1997;6: 557–65.
35. Flament JB, Delattre JF, Pluot M. Arterial blood supply to the parathyroid glands: Implications for thyroid surgery. Anat Clin 1982;3(3):279–87.
36. Delattre JF, Flament JB, Palot JP, et al. [Variations in the parathyroid glands. Number, situation and arterial vascularization. Anatomical study and surgical application]. J Chir 1982;119(11):633–41.
37. Jiang H, Shen H, Jiang D, et al. Evaluating the safety of the Harmonic Scalpel around the recurrent laryngeal nerve. ANZ J Surg 2010;80(11):822–6.
38. Papavramidis TS, Pliakos I, Chorti A, et al. Comparing LigasureTM Exact dissector with other energy devices in total thyroidectomy: a pilot study. Gland Surg 2020;9(2):271–7.
39. Promberger R, Ott J, Kober F, et al. Intra- and postoperative parathyroid hormone-kinetics do not advocate for autotransplantation of discolored parathyroid glands during thyroidectomy. Thyroid Off J Am Thyroid Assoc 2010;20(12): 1371–5.
40. Promberger R, Ott J, Bures C, et al. Can a surgeon predict the risk of postoperative hypoparathyroidism during thyroid surgery? A prospective study on self-assessment by experts. Am J Surg 2014;208(1):13–20.
41. Paras C, Keller M, Mahadevan-Jansen A, et al. Near-infrared autofluorescence for the detection of parathyroid glands. J Biomed Opt 2011;16(6):067012.
42. Solórzano CC, Thomas G, Berber E, et al. Current state of intraoperative use of near infrared fluorescence for parathyroid identification and preservation. Surgery 2021;169(4):868–78.
43. De Leeuw: Intraoperative near-infrared imaging for - Google Scholar. https://scholar.google.com/scholar_lookup?title=Intraoperative%20near-infrared%20imaging%20for%20parathyroid%20gland%20identification%20by%20auto-fluorescence%3A%20a%20feasibility%20study&publication_year=2016&author=F.%20De%20Leeuw&author=I.%20Breuskin&author=M.%20Abbaci. Accessed July 2, 2023.

44. McWade MA, Paras C, White LM, et al. Label-free Intraoperative Parathyroid Localization With Near-Infrared Autofluorescence Imaging. J Clin Endocrinol Metab 2014;99(12):4574–80.
45. McWade MA, Sanders ME, Broome JT, et al. Establishing the clinical utility of autofluorescence spectroscopy for parathyroid detection. Surgery 2016;159(1):193–203.
46. De Leeuw F, Breuskin I, Abbaci M, et al. Intraoperative Near-infrared Imaging for Parathyroid Gland Identification by Auto-fluorescence: A Feasibility Study. World J Surg 2016;40(9):2131–8.
47. McWade MA, Thomas G, Nguyen JQ, et al. Enhancing Parathyroid Gland Visualization Using a Near Infrared Fluorescence-Based Overlay Imaging System. J Am Coll Surg 2019;228(5):730–43.
48. Kose E, Kahramangil B, Aydin H, et al. Heterogeneous and low-intensity parathyroid autofluorescence: Patterns suggesting hyperfunction at parathyroid exploration. Surgery 2019;165(2):431–7.
49. DiMarco A, Chotalia R, Bloxham R, et al. Autofluorescence in Parathyroidectomy: Signal Intensity Correlates with Serum Calcium and Parathyroid Hormone but Routine Clinical Use is Not Justified. World J Surg 2019;43(6):1532–7.
50. Dip F, Falco J, Verna S, et al. Randomized Controlled Trial Comparing White Light with Near-Infrared Autofluorescence for Parathyroid Gland Identification During Total Thyroidectomy. J Am Coll Surg 2019;228(5):744–51.
51. Squires MH, Jarvis R, Shirley LA, et al. Intraoperative Parathyroid Autofluorescence Detection in Patients with Primary Hyperparathyroidism. Ann Surg Oncol 2019;26(4):1142–8.
52. Thomas G, McWade MA, Nguyen JQ, et al. Innovative surgical guidance for label-free real-time parathyroid identification. Surgery 2019;165(1):114–23.
53. Kim Y, Kim SW, Lee KD, et al. Real-time localization of the parathyroid gland in surgical field using Raspberry Pi during thyroidectomy: a preliminary report. Biomed Opt Express 2018;9(7):3391–8.
54. Alesina PF, Meier B, Hinrichs J, et al. Enhanced visualization of parathyroid glands during video-assisted neck surgery. Langenbeck's Arch Surg 2018;403(3):395–401.
55. Kahramangil B, Berber E. Comparison of indocyanine green fluorescence and parathyroid autofluorescence imaging in the identification of parathyroid glands during thyroidectomy. Gland Surg 2017;6(6):644–8.
56. Kim SW, Lee HS, Ahn YC, et al. Near-Infrared Autofluorescence Image-Guided Parathyroid Gland Mapping in Thyroidectomy. J Am Coll Surg 2018;226(2):165–72.
57. Benmiloud F, Rebaudet S, Varoquaux A, et al. Impact of autofluorescence-based identification of parathyroids during total thyroidectomy on postoperative hypocalcemia: a before and after controlled study. Surgery 2018;163(1):23–30.
58. Ladurner R, Sommerey S, Arabi NA, et al. Intraoperative near-infrared autofluorescence imaging of parathyroid glands. Surg Endosc 2017;31(8):3140–5.
59. Ladurner R, Al Arabi N, Guendogar U, et al. Near-infrared autofluorescence imaging to detect parathyroid glands in thyroid surgery. Ann R Coll Surg Engl 2018;100(1):33–6.
60. Falco J, Dip F, Quadri P, et al. Cutting Edge in Thyroid Surgery: Autofluorescence of Parathyroid Glands. J Am Coll Surg 2016;223(2):374–80.
61. Kim SW, Song SH, Lee HS, et al. Intraoperative Real-Time Localization of Normal Parathyroid Glands With Autofluorescence Imaging. J Clin Endocrinol Metab 2016;101(12):4646–52.

62. Obongo Anga R, Abbaci M, Guerlain J, et al. Intraoperative Autofluorescence Imaging for Parathyroid Gland Identification during Total Laryngectomy with Thyroidectomy. Cancers 2023;15(3):875.

63. Abe K, Takahashi T, Yokoyama Y, et al. Near-infrared autofluorescence identification of ectopic parathyroid lesions. Laryngoscope 2023. https://doi.org/10.1002/lary.30728.

64. Sehnem L, Noureldine SI, Avci S, et al. A multicenter evaluation of near-infrared autofluorescence imaging of parathyroid glands in thyroid and parathyroid surgery. Surgery 2023;173(1):132–7.

65. Huang J, He Y, Wang Y, et al. Prevention of hypoparathyroidism: A step-by-step near-infrared autofluorescence parathyroid identification method. Front Endocrinol 2023;14:1086367.

66. Falco J, Dip F, Quadri P, et al. Increased identification of parathyroid glands using near infrared light during thyroid and parathyroid surgery. Surg Endosc 2017;31(9):3737–42.

67. Barbieri D, Indelicato P, Vinciguerra A, et al. Autofluorescence and Indocyanine Green in Thyroid Surgery: A Systematic Review and Meta-Analysis. Laryngoscope 2021;131(7):1683–92.

68. Rudin AV, McKenzie TJ, Thompson GB, et al. Evaluation of Parathyroid Glands with Indocyanine Green Fluorescence Angiography After Thyroidectomy. World J Surg 2019;43(6):1538–43.

69. Triponez F. Re: Evaluation of Parathyroid Glands with Indocyanine Green Fluorescence Angiography After Thyroidectomy. World J Surg 2019;43(6):1544–5.

70. Vidal Fortuny J, Sadowski SM, Belfontali V, et al. Randomized clinical trial of intraoperative parathyroid gland angiography with indocyanine green fluorescence predicting parathyroid function after thyroid surgery. Br J Surg 2018;105(4):350–7.

71. Zaidi N, Bucak E, Yazici P, et al. The feasibility of indocyanine green fluorescence imaging for identifying and assessing the perfusion of parathyroid glands during total thyroidectomy. J Surg Oncol 2016;113(7):775–8.

72. Gálvez-Pastor S, Torregrosa NM, Ríos A, et al. Prediction of hypocalcemia after total thyroidectomy using indocyanine green angiography of parathyroid glands: A simple quantitative scoring system. Am J Surg 2019;218(5):993–9.

73. Jin H, Dong Q, He Z, et al. Research on indocyanine green angiography for predicting postoperative hypoparathyroidism. Clin Endocrinol 2019;90(3):487–93.

74. Sadowski SM, Vidal Fortuny J, Triponez F. A reappraisal of vascular anatomy of the parathyroid gland based on fluorescence techniques. Gland Surg 2017;6(Suppl 1):S30–7.

75. Benmiloud F, Penaranda G, Chiche L, et al. Intraoperative Mapping Angiograms of the Parathyroid Glands Using Indocyanine Green During Thyroid Surgery: Results of the Fluogreen Study. World J Surg 2022;46(2):416–24.

Avoiding Complications of Thyroidectomy

Recurrent Laryngeal Nerve and Superior Laryngeal Nerve Preservation

Kevin Y. Liang, MD, Joseph Scharpf, MD*

KEYWORDS

- Thyroidectomy • Recurrent laryngeal nerve • Superior laryngeal nerve

KEY POINTS

- Recurrent laryngeal nerve injury during thyroidectomy is rare but can have significant morbidity.
- The superior laryngeal nerve is also at risk during thyroidectomy and has highly variable anatomy.
- Thorough preoperative history, physical examination, and review of imaging are crucial.
- Exposing the nerves is the safest way to protect them.

INTRODUCTION

A dreaded complication of thyroid surgery is injury to the recurrent laryngeal nerve (RLN). A systematic review including more than 25,000 patients estimated the incidence rate of temporary and permanent RLN palsy after thyroidectomy to be 9.8% and 2.3%, respectively.[1] Fortunately, RLN injury rates from thyroidectomy have decreased to the point that nonthyroid surgeries (eg, anterior approach to the cervical spine, carotid endarterectomy) are now the most common iatrogenic cause.[2] However, thyroidectomy is still the most common cause of iatrogenic bilateral vocal fold immobility.[2] RLN injury can result in significant dysphonia and/or dysphagia, although sometimes patients with a vocal fold paresis can have remarkably normal voice and swallow function.[3]

Another less commonly discussed complication of thyroidectomy is injury to the superior laryngeal nerve (SLN). The external branch provides motor innervation to the cricothyroid muscle, which tenses the vocal fold and elevates pitch. Injury rates

Head and Neck Institute, Cleveland Clinic Foundation, 9500 Euclid Avenue, A71, Cleveland, OH 44195, USA
* Corresponding author.
E-mail address: Scharpj@ccf.org

Otolaryngol Clin N Am 57 (2024) 75–82
https://doi.org/10.1016/j.otc.2023.08.001
0030-6665/24/© 2023 Elsevier Inc. All rights reserved.

oto.theclinics.com

in the literature vary widely and can be up to 58%.[4–6] Less is known about SLN injuries perhaps because the clinical manifestations are more subtle. In this article, we provide a comprehensive preoperative and intraoperative guide to preserving both the RLN and SLN during thyroid surgery.

PREOPERATIVE EVALUATION

Preservation of the RLN and SLN begins not at the time of surgery but during the initial patient evaluation. It is the senior author's routine practice to perform subjective and objective evaluation of vocal fold function before any planned thyroid surgery. A careful history is taken, especially for any voice or swallow complaint. Any prior skull base, neck, or chest surgery is noted, including the laterality. Vocal fold movement is assessed with laryngoscopy—either through indirect mirror examination or through flexible laryngoscopy. Any preoperative vocal fold immobility or hypomobility can influence the surgical plan during thyroidectomy. Preoperative vocal fold assessment admittedly may not always be feasible. The American Academy of Otolaryngology (AAO) Clinical Practice Guideline: Improving Voice Outcomes after Thyroid Surgery recommends vocal fold mobility assessment if there is existing vocal impairment or if the voice is normal but the patient has either thyroid cancer with suspected extrathyroidal extension or earlier surgery that increases the risk of RLN injury.[7]

Preoperative imaging with ultrasound and possibly cross-sectional imaging can be of great value in alerting the surgeon to the anatomic location of the nerves based on the thyroid shape and size. Furthermore, an aberrant subclavian artery on the right side, which generally can be readily appreciated via ultrasound or cross-sectional imaging (**Fig. 1**) can preoperatively alert the surgeon to the presence of a non-RLN.

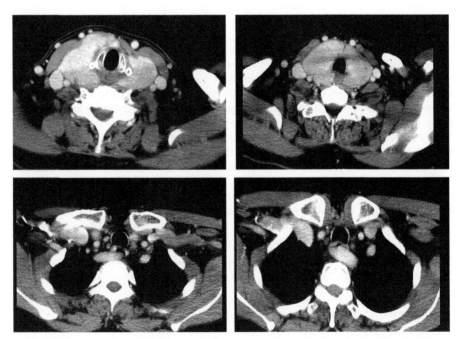

Fig. 1. Aberrant right subclavian artery with nonrecurrent right laryngeal nerve appreciated intraoperatively.

This proactive preoperative assessment could certainly aid in the anatomic intraoperative dissection.

The indications for surgery are also crucial for operative planning. Inflammatory diseases (eg, Hashimoto thyroiditis) or large goiters can potentially displace the RLN and SLN from their typical locations. The pathologic condition will also dictate the extent of surgery. If a central neck dissection is planned for malignancy, a greater segment of the RLN must be dissected free. The patient should be counseled preoperatively on possible RLN sacrifice if there is already clinical suspicion of nerve invasion or encasement.

GENERAL OPERATIVE PRINCIPLES TO AVOID NERVE INJURY

Meticulous hemostasis throughout the thyroidectomy is of utmost importance. This provides the surgeon with the optimal view to identify critical landmarks that lead to identifying the nerves. This process is greatly aided when the tissue is not blood-stained. In many instances, simple direct pressure with a gauze will stop most low-volume oozing. When bleeding must be controlled, the authors advocate for precise bipolar cautery, surgical clips, or suture tying rather than monopolar cautery. Advanced energy devices are also frequently used and seem to be quite effective in thyroid surgery.[8,9] Additionally, keeping dissection directly on the thyroid capsule will minimize injury risk to nerves as well as parathyroid glands and other surrounding tissue. In addition to precise anatomic dissection and hemostasis without heat injury to the nerve, careful awareness of maintaining minimal traction on a very delicate RLN (**Fig. 2**) is of utmost importance.

INTRAOPERATIVE NEURAL MONITORING

The routine use of intraoperative neural monitoring (IONM) in thyroid surgery has become more common, particularly among high volume surgeons.[10,11] A common method of nerve monitoring is through an electromyographic system using a specialized endotracheal tube with bilateral electrodes to monitor laryngeal musculature activation. The alert system can be activated through nerve pressure, heat, traction, or intentional stimulation with a probe. One drawback of IONM use is cost of the additional equipment, adding approximately 5% to 7% to a thyroidectomy.[12] Additionally, IONM has some inherent risk of false positives and negatives, which could affect surgical confidence and operating time. However, there are several benefits to IONM. The surgeon can identify the RLN and map its course along the paratracheal region. The RLN can be detected in nearly 100% of cases with IONM.[10] One prospective,

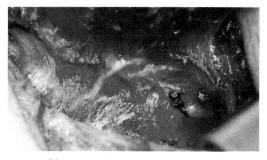

Fig. 2. Delicate RLN susceptible to traction injury.

randomized study demonstrated a nearly 3-fold reduction in time to identify the RLN when using IONM.[11] An additional benefit of IONM is providing prognostication regarding RLN function. Final intraoperative evoked potential amplitudes strongly correlate with immediate postoperative vocal fold function.[13] This is especially valuable when considering staging the contralateral lobectomy to prevent possible airway compromise if both RLNs were either temporarily or permanently injured. Although there are limitations to IONM, the senior author and the International Neural Monitoring Study Group support its routine use in thyroid surgery.[10] At a minimum, the AAO recommends that surgeons consider IONM for bilateral thyroid surgery, revision thyroid surgery, and surgery in the setting of an existing RLN paralysis.[7]

RECURRENT LARYNGEAL NERVE

The RLN comes off of the vagus nerve and runs around the aortic arch on the left side and the subclavian artery on the right. The nerve runs in the tracheoesophageal groove (more laterally on the right), passing deep to the inferior pharyngeal constrictor muscle and posterior to the cricothyroid joint to enter the larynx. The nerve provides both sensation to the glottis and subglottis and motor innervation to all intrinsic laryngeal muscles except the cricothyroid. Before the 1900s, it was a commonplace for surgeons to try minimizing nerve injury by intentionally avoiding the nerve. However, multiple surgeons in the early twentieth century demonstrated that the RLN could routinely be identified and preserved during thyroid surgery.[14,15] More contemporary data have further endorsed the notion that identifying the RLN results in fewer nerve injuries.[16]

There are multiple strategies to identify the RLN. An inferolateral approach described by Loré involves finding the nerve in the tracheoesophageal groove through careful blunt dissection within a triangle bounded by the trachea and esophagus medially, the carotid artery laterally, and the inferior thyroid pole superiorly.[17] Simon described a similar triangle bounded by the carotid artery laterally, the esophagus medially, and the inferior thyroid artery superiorly.[18] The RLN is most often deep to the inferior thyroid artery but can be superficial to or branch around the artery.[3,19] The RLN can also be identified more superiorly because it enters the larynx. Because the cricoid cartilage is a very easily palpable landmark, the nerve can usually be quickly identified through blunt dissection posterior to the cricothyroid joint. Careful attention must be given to any potential branching of the nerve before entering the larynx. The tubercle of Zuckerkandl, a remnant of the ultimobranchial body, is also a useful landmark because the RLN typically runs posterior and medial to the tubercle.[20]

A rare variant of the RLN (0.7% prevalence) is a non-RLN, resulting in a much more horizontal course than is typical.[21] A non-RLN is usually on the right side and is associated with an aberrant subclavian artery in the vast majority (87%) of cases.[21] Preoperatively, the surgeon should keep suspicion high for this anomaly if the patient is found to have a retro-esophageal subclavian artery (see **Fig. 1**) causing dysphagia lusoria. The senior author routinely performs ultrasound in clinic preoperatively, thus identifying any abnormal anatomy that would suggest non-RLN. If ultrasound was not completed ahead of time, a preincision ultrasound can be performed in the operating room. Intraoperatively, if the RLN is not found in the tracheoesophageal groove, one must be very careful dissecting laterally because the exact trajectory of the nerve will be unpredictable.

SUPERIOR LARYNGEAL NERVE

Although RLN injury is a well-known complication of thyroid surgery, the SLN is also at risk. The SLN comes off of the vagus nerve and divides into internal and external branches. The internal branch runs with the superior laryngeal artery through the thyrohyoid membrane to provide sensation to the supraglottic and glottis. The internal branch is uncommonly encountered during thyroid surgery given its proximal entry point into the larynx. The external branch of the superior laryngeal nerve (EBSLN) provides motor innervation to the cricothyroid muscle, which causes pitch elevation by tensing the vocal fold (**Fig. 3**). The course of the nerve is classically variable, and there have been multiple classification systems developed to account for the anatomic deviations. The Cernea classification[22,23] is based on the where the nerve crosses the superior thyroid artery in relation to the superior thyroid pole (**Fig. 4**). The most dangerous presentation of the EBSLN is over the gland, a Cernea Type IIb classification. The Friedman classification[24] is based on whether the nerve runs superficial, through, or deep to the inferior pharyngeal constrictor muscle.

When dissecting at the superior pole, one must stay as close to the thyroid capsule as possible. The superior thyroid vessels should be divided close to the thyroid to minimize the risk to the EBSLN. Moreover, given the anatomic variability of the EBSLN, the authors recommend nerve preservation by direct identification whenever feasible. When the nerve is unable to be located, careful attention should be paid to exclude the nerve's presence when dividing tissue at the superior pole. This can be accomplished visually or with nerve monitoring. Cernea concluded in a randomized prospective trial

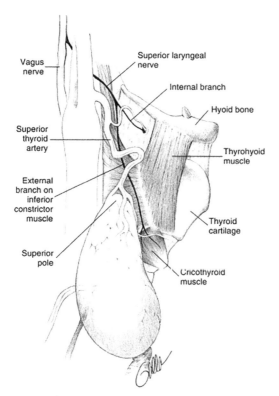

Fig. 3. The EBSLN descends from the vagus nerve behind the internal and external carotid arteries and courses medially to the larynx. (*With permission from* Gregory W. Randolph, MD, FACS, FACE, FEBS (Endocrine), MAMSE. Randolph GW (ed) Surgery of the Thyroid and Parathyroid Glands. 3rd edition Philadelphia, PA: Elsevier Saunders, 2020 ISBN:978-0-323-66127-0.)

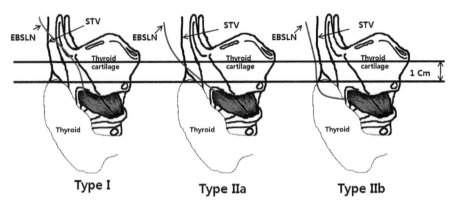

Fig. 4. Cernea's classification based on where the EBSLN crosses the superior thyroid vessels in relation to the superior thyroid pole. STV, superior thyroid vessels; EBSLN, exterior branch of the superior laryngeal nerve. (*From* Hwang SB, Lee HY, Kim WY, et al. The anatomy of the external branch of the superior laryngeal nerve in Koreans. Asian J Surg. Jan 2013;36(1):13 to 9. https://doi.org/10.1016/j.asjsur.2012.08.003, with permission.)

that even in his own hands, careful dissection of the superior pole without EBSLN identification leads to significantly more nerve injuries than when the nerve is identified with a nerve stimulator.[22] Additionally, a systematic review and meta-analysis of over 13,000 hemilarynges concluded that IONM improves EBSLN identification rates.[25]

CLINICS CARE POINTS

- Comprehensive preoperative evaluation is paramount for surgical planning.
- The RLN is often times found either in the tracheoesophageal groove from an inferolateral approach or more superiorly before it enters the larynx.
- The external branch of the SLN has highly variable anatomy. Dissecting out the superior pole must be performed methodically to avoid injuring this nerve.
- IONM can be very beneficial in identifying and preserving both the RLN and SLN.

DISCLOSURE

The authors do not have any funding sources or conflicts of interest to disclose.

REFERENCES

1. Serpell JW, Lee JC, Yeung MJ, et al. Differential recurrent laryngeal nerve palsy rates after thyroidectomy. Surgery 2014;156(5):1157–66.
2. Rosenthal LH, Benninger MS, Deeb RH. Vocal fold immobility: a longitudinal analysis of etiology over 20 years. Laryngoscope 2007;117(10):1864–70.
3. Benninger MS, Scharpf J. Vocal Fold Paralysis and Thyroid Surgery. In: Hanks JB, Inabnet WB, editors. Controversies in thyroid surgery. Springer International Publishing; 2016. p. 109–23.
4. Jansson S, Tisell LE, Hagne I, et al. Partial superior laryngeal nerve (SLN) lesions before and after thyroid surgery. World J Surg 1988;12(4):522–7.

5. Teitelbaum BJ, Wenig BL. Superior laryngeal nerve injury from thyroid surgery. Head Neck 1995;17(1):36–40.

6. Stojadinovic A, Shaha AR, Orlikoff RF, et al. Prospective functional voice assessment in patients undergoing thyroid surgery. Ann Surg 2002;236(6):823–32.

7. Chandrasekhar SS, Randolph GW, Seidman MD, et al. Clinical practice guideline: improving voice outcomes after thyroid surgery. Otolaryngol Head Neck Surg 2013;148(6 Suppl):S1–37.

8. Manouras A, Markogiannakis HE, Kekis PB, et al. Novel hemostatic devices in thyroid surgery: electrothermal bipolar vessel sealing system and harmonic scalpel. Expert Rev Med Devices 2008;5(4):447 66.

9. Miccoli P, Berti P, Dionigi G, et al. Randomized controlled trial of harmonic scalpel use during thyroidectomy. Arch Otolaryngol Head Neck Surg 2006;132(10): 1069–73.

10. Randolph GW, Dralle H, Abdullah H, et al. Electrophysiologic recurrent laryngeal nerve monitoring during thyroid and parathyroid surgery: international standards guideline statement. Laryngoscope 2011;121(Suppl 1):S1–16.

11. Sarı S, Erbil Y, Sümer A, et al. Evaluation of recurrent laryngeal nerve monitoring in thyroid surgery. Int J Surg 2010;8(6):474–8.

12. Dionigi G, Bacuzzi A, Boni L, et al. Visualization versus neuromonitoring of recurrent laryngeal nerves during thyroidectomy: what about the costs? World J Surg 2012;36(4):748–54.

13. Genther DJ, Kandil EH, Noureldine SI, et al. Correlation of final evoked potential amplitudes on intraoperative electromyography of the recurrent laryngeal nerve with immediate postoperative vocal fold function after thyroid and parathyroid surgery. JAMA Otolaryngol Head Neck Surg 2014;140(2):124–8.

14. Lahey FH, Hoover WB. Injuries to the recurrent laryngeal nerve in thyroid operations: their management and avoidance. Ann Surg 1938;108(4):545–62.

15. RIDDELL VH. Injury to recurrent laryngeal nerves during thyroidectomy; a comparison between the results of identification and non-identification in 1022 nerves exposed to risk. Lancet 1956;271(6944):638–41.

16. Hermann M, Alk G, Roka R, et al. Laryngeal recurrent nerve injury in surgery for benign thyroid diseases: effect of nerve dissection and impact of individual surgeon in more than 27,000 nerves at risk. Ann Surg 2002;235(2):261–8.

17. Loré JM, Kim DJ, Elias S. Preservation of the laryngeal nerves during total thyroid lobectomy. Ann Otol Rhinol Laryngol 1977;86(6 Pt 1):777–88.

18. SIMON MM. Safeguarding the recurrent laryngeal nerve in thyroid surgery: a triangle for its localization and protection. Miss Valley Med J 1957;79(4): 180–6.

19. Ngo Nyeki AR, Njock LR, Miloundja J, et al. Recurrent laryngeal nerve landmarks during thyroidectomy. Eur Ann Otorhinolaryngol Head Neck Dis 2015;132(5): 265–9.

20. Gauger PG, Delbridge LW, Thompson NW, et al. Incidence and importance of the tubercle of Zuckerkandl in thyroid surgery. Eur J Surg 2001;167(4):249–54.

21. Henry BM, Sanna S, Graves MJ, et al. The Non-Recurrent Laryngeal Nerve: a meta-analysis and clinical considerations. PeerJ 2017;5:e3012.

22. Cernea CR, Ferraz AR, Furlani J, et al. Identification of the external branch of the superior laryngeal nerve during thyroidectomy. Am J Surg 1992;164(6): 634–9.

23. Cernea CR, Ferraz AR, Nishio S, et al. Surgical anatomy of the external branch of the superior laryngeal nerve. Head Neck 1992;14(5):380–3.

24. Friedman M, LoSavio P, Ibrahim H. Superior laryngeal nerve identification and preservation in thyroidectomy. Arch Otolaryngol Head Neck Surg 2002;128(3): 296–303.
25. Cheruiyot I, Kipkorir V, Henry BM, et al. Surgical anatomy of the external branch of the superior laryngeal nerve: a systematic review and meta-analysis. Langenbeck's Arch Surg 2018;403(7):811–23.

Radiofrequency Ablation for Benign Nodules and for Cancer, Too?

Jonathon O. Russell, MD, FACS*, Kaitlyn M. Frazier, MD

KEYWORDS

- Radiofrequency ablation • Benign thyroid nodules • Symptomatic thyroid nodules
- Papillary thyroid carcinoma • Thyroid cancer quality of life

KEY POINTS

- Radiofrequency ablation (RFA) is a minimally invasive technique that can be performed in an outpatient or clinic setting and offers the ability to improve compressive and cosmetic symptoms from thyroid nodules with minimal down time and a low complication rate.
- Surgery remains the recommendation for thyroid cancer and autonomous functioning nodules in most circumstances, although RFA may offer an alternative to active surveillance for very low-risk cancers or treatment of very limited recurrent cancer.
- The role of RFA in autonomous functioning nodules, thyroid cancer, and indeterminate nodules is controversial and remains an area of investigation.

BACKGROUND

Historical Perspective

One of the earliest descriptions of procedures to treat thyroid disease came from Roger Frugardii in Salerno, Italy in 1170 CE: he described an operation that involved the insertion of heated iron setons into a thyroid mass and serial manipulation until they broke the skin surface.[1,2] During the next millennium, innumerable advancements in surgical techniques and safety established open thyroidectomy as the standard of care for symptomatic or malignant nodules. Now, almost 1000 years after Frugardii, transcutaneous thermal ablation of thyroid masses is experiencing a twenty-first century renaissance.

Percutaneous radiofrequency ablation (RFA) is the most widely adopted thermal technique for thyroid nodules. Initially used for the treatment of inoperable liver lesions, an early case series of 8 patients in 2001 applied RFA for ablation of regional recurrences from well-differentiated thyroid cancer.[3] RFA for benign thyroid nodules

Department of Otolaryngology–Head & Neck Surgery, Johns Hopkins University School of Medicine, 601 North Caroline Street, 6th Floor, Baltimore, MD 21287, USA
* Corresponding author.
E-mail address: jrusse41@jhmi.edu

Otolaryngol Clin N Am 57 (2024) 83–97
https://doi.org/10.1016/j.otc.2023.09.004
0030-6665/24/© 2023 Elsevier Inc. All rights reserved.

oto.theclinics.com

(BTNs) was first described in small cohorts in 2006 in Korea[4] and in 2007 in Italy[5] with promising results. A series of 302 benign nodules treated by Jeong and colleagues in 2008 demonstrated (1) efficacy with a mean nodule volume reduction ratio (VRR) of 84% and (2) safety with no long-lasting complications (short-term complications included pain, hematoma, and 3 patients with transient hoarseness of less than 2 months).[6]

Thyroid applications of RFA continued to gain popularity in Asia, with the first guidelines for use introduced by the Korean Society of Thyroid Radiology in 2009 (last revised in 2017).[7,8] A 2015 randomized trial treating benign nodules with the "moving shot" RFA technique further established the efficacy of RFA with a mean nodule volume reduction of 71%, as well as improvement of patient scores for subjective compressive and cosmetic symptoms.[9] In 2018, the Food Drug Administration (FDA) approved an RFA device designed for thyroid ablation in the United States, the same year as the first US case series for benign nodules was published.[10] The European Thyroid Association established clinical practice guidelines for minimally invasive ablation treatment of benign (2020)[11] and malignant (2021)[12] thyroid nodules. More recently, a 2022 consortium of major endocrine and surgical societies synthesized an international consensus statement for the use of RFA for both benign and malignant thyroid lesions.[13]

Mechanism of Action

RFA achieves tissue coagulation necrosis via thermal energy, with resultant volume reduction in thyroid nodules over the following months. The electrode needle is introduced into the target nodule under ultrasound guidance, and an electrical current is applied to the nodule. The alternating current creates tissue ionic agitation and resultant frictional heat, resulting in local thermal coagulation necrosis once temperatures of 60°C to 100°C are reached (the premise of the "moving shot" repositioning technique detailed below).[14,15] Slightly lower temperatures of 50°C cause irreversible tissue damage if sustained during 4 to 6 minutes. The treatment effect has the highest density in the tissue zone adjacent to the electrode but tissue that is further away is also ablated slowly via thermal conduction. The electrode is internally cooled with normal saline infused by a peristaltic pump, which prevents char at the electrode surface and thus increases energy transfer to surrounding tissues.

DISCUSSION
Indications, Preprocedural Evaluation, and Counseling

RFA is FDA approved in the United States for percutaneous and intraoperative coagulation and ablation of tissue. A device marketed for thyroid ablation was approved in 2018. Standard workup for a thyroid nodule should be performed, including thyroid ultrasound, fine needle aspiration biopsy (FNAB), and thyroid function testing. Guidelines generally recommend 2 benign biopsies for treatment, with an exception for spongiform nodules that are very low suspicion (**Fig. 1**).[8,11,13,16,17]

Benign nodules

RFA is offered for compressive or cosmetic concerns associated with BTNs—the recommended practice is to treat the patient and their symptoms, not the presence of the nodule.[13] Patients may prefer RFA over thyroidectomy for many reasons, from a desire to avoid surgical recovery, desire to avoid a scar if scarless surgery is not available in their area, high value placed on preserving thyroid function, or comorbid conditions that increase the surgical risk.[11,13,16,18] Some guidelines suggest a size of 20 to 30 mm in largest diameter as a minimum for recommending RFA,[11] although smaller

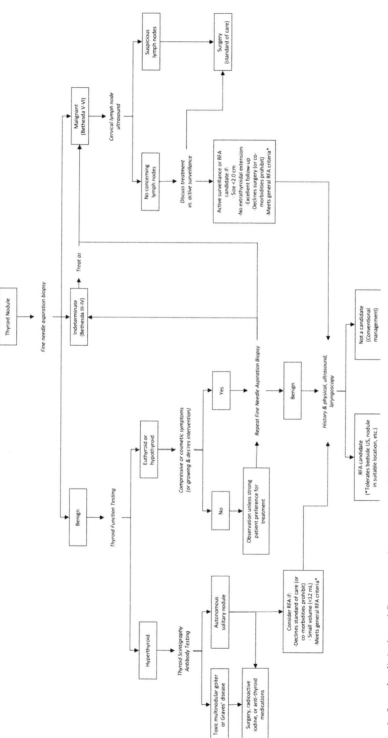

Fig. 1. Sample clinical workflow to evaluate RFA candidacy for benign, indeterminate, malignant, and functioning thyroid nodules.

nodules may be symptomatic based on location and patient body habitus and there-fore appropriate for treatment.[13] A history of growth may also support treatment. There is no defined upper size limit for the treatment of BTNs, although larger nodules may still be large and symptomatic even if they are reduced in volume by 50% (the standard definition of successful response) or may require multiple treatments. Patient symptoms may be quantified by quality-of-life scales such as the Thyroid-Related Patient-Reported Outcome (ThyPRO or abbreviated ThyPRO-39), Short Form Health Survey, simple symptom visual analog scales, and clinician ratings. Given that compressive or cosmetic concerns represent the most common procedural indica-tion, documentation of a measurable baseline for these complaints may establish benefit from RFA. The 2022 international consensus statement supports the use of patient-reported outcomes to determine efficacy.[13]

Is my patient a candidate?

Workup for RFA candidacy also includes a full head and neck examination including flexible laryngoscopy and an ultrasound by the primary treatment team. During phys-ical examination, particular attention should be paid to neck landmarks, girth, length, range of motion, and tolerance of supine position. In addition to screening for preex-isting cranial neuropathies, preprocedure laryngoscopy is performed to establish a patient-specific baseline in the event of a temporary paresis. Others use transcuta-neous laryngeal sonography for the same purpose, although older age (>70 years), male gender, tall body height, obese body habitus, and calcified thyroid cartilage make laryngeal sonography more challenging.[19]

Preprocedure ultrasonography by the treatment team is essential to understanding eligibility and likelihood of success, as well as anticipate intraprocedural difficulties, of RFA for a particular patient. Certain nodule locations carry higher risks. Of greatest note is the "danger triangle,"—the interface between the posteromedial thyroid lobe, trachea, and esophagus where the recurrent laryngeal nerve is expected to lie.[15] However, other nodule locations are also at higher risk of complications or of reduced ability to treat: tracheal adjacent, retrocarotid, and substernal.

Technique

Prerequisite skills include ultrasonography and FNAB experience. Equipment includes a procedural quality ultrasound machine, radiofrequency (RF) generator, and RF elec-trode. Electrodes are available in active tip lengths ranging from 3 to 15 mm—we use 10 to 15-mm probes for most benign disease and 5-mm probes for malignancy or small benign nodules in sensitive areas requiring more precise energy delivery.

Procedural best practices

The procedure is performed under local anesthesia. Generous infiltration of local anes-thetic is key to patient tolerance of the procedure. Best practice is to reach the nodule via a "transisthmic approach."[20] If the nodule is adjacent to a structure that should remain sensate, dextrose 5% solution (a nonionic, isotonic solution) may be infused for both hydrodissection to create separation and to serve as a heat sink.[13,21,22] The dextrose solution may be infused either intermittently via a needle and syringe or continuously via an angiocatheter. We encourage the patient to talk throughout the procedure, which allows monitoring of any early vocal changes, and to inform us of increased heat sensation or pain.

Multiple passes of the electrode needle visualized in the long axis are used to deliver energy throughout the nodule, a continuous repositioning, which is known as the "moving shot" technique.[9,15] The general concept is to start with a trajectory toward the deep and medial aspect of the nodule and treat as the needle is withdrawn. The initial starting point is critical because superficial treatment early in the procedure will create sonographic artifact that makes it more difficult to treat the deeper areas. The nodule is divided into "conceptual ablation units" (**Fig. 2**).[20] Ablation radius depends on electrode active tip length and time; accordingly, conceptual unit size can be tailored based on location within the nodule. Nodule tissue near the danger triangle or critical structures should be treated with smaller conceptual units, erring toward undertreatment if needed. Ablated tissue will begin to appear hyperechoic, and impedances should be monitored for an increase to indicate tissue necrosis has occurred. The electrode is then repositioned and sequential treatment of conceptual ablation units continues.

We typically start treatment at 45 W for midsized benign and 5 to 15 W for malignant nodules, and uptitrate power if hyperechoic changes are not seen within 5 to 10 seconds.[15] Lower power may be used around critical structures or if the patient experiences discomfort, and higher power is used with larger active needle tip length. Throughout treatment, particular attention should be paid to feeding blood vessels to limit their heat sink effects. Total energy delivered usually should reach 2000 J/mL for benign nodules, although this estimate is less accurate for very small or large nodules as volume changes are not linear. Increased energy delivery per unit volume has been associated with improved outcomes—Deandrea and colleagues cited a median energy of 1509 J/mL for nodules achieving VRR greater than 50%, and targets of 2109 and 2670 J/mL to achieve 95% and 99% probabilities of success—but it is not

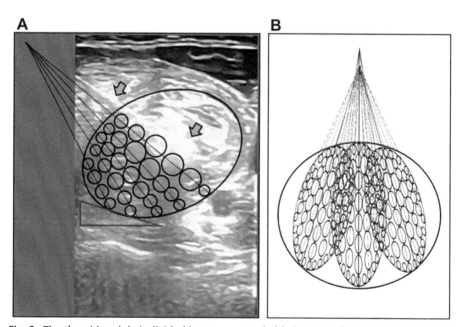

Fig. 2. The thyroid nodule is divided into conceptual ablation units for treatment. (*A*) Axial view of a transisthmic approach for a left-sided nodule (*danger triangle in red*). Schema of conceptual ablation units and needle trajectory (*black*) imposed on a thyroid nodule undergoing RFA treatment. Hyperechoic changes from RF electrode (*green arrows*) indicate successful ablation. Conceptual ablation unit size varies, with smaller sizes near periphery and adjacent to danger triangle. (*B*) Schema of multiple completed axial treatments at various longitudinal positions along nodule.

clear if there is a maximum level above which complications such as nodule rupture are more likely to occur.[23]

Postprocedure laryngoscopy is performed if there is a subjective voice change during treatment and considered if there is intent to treat the contralateral side. Sonographic evaluation of the larynx may be valuable as an immediately available adjunct. It should be noted that delayed voice changes and presumed palsies have been anecdotally reported; concurrent bilateral nodule treatment should therefore be approached with great caution.

Outcomes for Benign Nodules

RFA is associated with meaningful nodule volume reduction for BTNs. The technical definition of success is a VRR of more than 50% (VRR is defined as [Initial volume – posttreatment volume]/initial volume × 100, expressed as a percentage.) The majority of studies show a VRR greater than 70%, and patients that respond to RFA may continue to have nodule shrinkage (additional 10%–20% reduction) at a year or more after treatment.[24–28] Patients are typically followed with postprocedure thyroid function tests, and repeat thyroid ultrasounds at a minimum of 3, 6, and 12 months, and then followed thereafter as per their routine nodule surveillance protocol.[8,11,13,29]

A recent large multicenter, prospective cohort North American study demonstrated effectiveness in BTNs in the United States patient population.[30] The investigators enrolled 233 patients; mean greatest initial nodule diameter was 2.73 cm (interquartile range [IQR] 1.58–4.22) and volume of 4.17 mL (IQR 0.74–17.90); VRR at 6 and 12 months was 73% (IQR 51–90) and 76% (IQR 52–90) respectively, achieved in the vast majority of patients (94%) with only a single-treatment session. There was no significant change in thyroid function laboratory tests at 1 month posttreatment, consistent with multiple international studies.

Factors influencing volume reduction

Initial size of the nodule has been suggested to be an important factor in predicting response to RFA. In a 5-year study of nodules undergoing a single RFA treatment session, Deandrea and colleagues demonstrated that small nodules (<10 mL) reach their ultimate VRR early in follow-up (mean VRRs: 6 months 79%, 1 year 78%, and 5 years 81.8%), medium nodules (≥10 to <20 mL) continue to have reduction up to 2 years but ultimately reach comparable reduction to small nodules (6 months 59%, 1 year 66.7%, 2 years 74.2%, and 5 years 74.5%), and larger nodules (≥20 mL) have lower overall VRR (6 months 54.5%, 1 year 60.9%, 2 years 62.4%, and 5 years 65.3%).[24] Lim and colleagues demonstrated similar size-dependent response both for VRR during 4 years but also for number of treatments required, with small nodules requiring an average of 1.7 treatments, medium nodules 2.8 treatments, and larger nodules 3.8 treatments.[25] Sim and colleagues and Li and colleagues found regrowth rates (defined as greater than 50% increase from smallest volume achieved) of 19% to 24.1%, with highest risk of regrowth occurring around 3 years (study follow-up periods of 5–7 years).[31,32] When regrowth occurred, it originated from an undertreated nodule periphery in larger nodules, emphasizing the importance of tailoring peripheral conceptual ablation units to minimize marginal regrowth. In addition to this evidence that larger nodules have less volume reduction and higher regrowth rates, very large nodules may still be unacceptably large and symptomatic nodule even if technical success (VRR >50%) is achieved.

Other than nodule size considerations, Deandrea and colleagues investigated preprocedural ultrasound features and RFA response, and noted some subtle but consistent trends. They observed that spongiform (microcystic) nodules had a better VRR of 76% compared with nodules with mixed solid and cystic (VRR 67%) or solid

(66%) composition.[33] Peripheral vascularity seems to predict a marginal decrease in volume reduction and is a factor that has been found to increase the risk of regrowth, providing another reason to treat supplying blood vessels beyond their heat sink effects.[32] Postprocedurally, nodules treated with RFA often present a radiological conundrum. Subsequent ultrasounds may demonstrate heterogeneity with hyperechoic and hypoechoic changes, calcifications, cystic areas, and ill-defined margins that must be interpreted in the context of ablation.[34]

Symptom reduction

Perhaps as importantly as reducing nodule volume, RFA reduces compressive and cosmetic symptom scores. A multi-institutional study found patient-rated compressive symptoms improved from a mean of 3.6/10 at baseline to 0.4/10 at 6 months posttreatment (where 0 = no symptoms and 10 = serious symptoms that affect quality of life), and physician-rated cosmetic scores improved from 3.6/4 at baseline to 1.7/4 at 6 months (where 1 = not palpable or visible, 2 = palpable but not visible, 3 = visible nearby or on swallowing, and 4 = readily detectable).[9] The previously described, larger and longer term studies from these groups demonstrated durable improvements in both these areas.[24,25]

Side effects and complication rates

The most common side effects from RFA treatment are neck soreness, bruising, and swelling. There is a small risk of transient hyperthyroidism that resolves by 1 month. Serious complications from RFA are rare but are similar in type (although not frequency) to thyroid surgery. Overall complication rates include transient (1.44%, literature range 0.5%–4.7%) or permanent (0.17%) voice change, hematoma (0.62%, literature range 0.62%–17%), vasovagal reaction (literature range 0.34%–2.5%), skin burn (0.29%), and nodule rupture (0.17%) without or with infection (0.08%), with case reports of brachial plexus injury and Horner syndrome.[35,36]

Autonomous Nodules

The vast majority of benign nodules are nonfunctioning but a patient found to have hyperthyroidism should undergo further workup which would inform possible eligibility for RFA (see **Fig. 1**). The presence of multiple foci of hyperactivity on scintigraphy or Graves disease suggests poor RFA candidacy. RFA is still viewed as a second-line treatment option even for solitary toxic autonomously functioning thyroid nodules (AFTNs) because the rate of enduring euthyroidism is lower for RFA than other management approaches.[37] Guidelines permit treatment of AFTNs with RFA as a safe therapeutic alternative if there are contraindications for first-line techniques.[13]

Rate of conversion to euthyroidism varies considerably across studies. A large meta-analysis found the pooled rate of euthyroidism after RFA for solitary AFTNs is 57%, much lower than for thyroidectomy, antithyroid drugs, or radioactive iodine.[37] Overall success generally seems to be size dependent—a smaller nodule initial volume (<12 mL) and achieving a posttreatment volume reduction of 80% correlate with achieving euthyroidism.[37,38] Cesareo and colleagues found that baseline volume represented the only significant predictor in achieving clinical response of euthyroidism (sex, age, and baseline thyroid-stimulating hormone were not correlated).[38] Dobnig and colleagues noted a significantly higher treatment energy required compared with nontoxic nodules (0.56 vs 0.35 kcal/mL, or 2343 vs 1464 J/mL) to achieve euthyroid results.[39]

Radiofrequency Ablation for Malignancy?

Although surgery remains the standard of care, multiple investigations of RFA for thyroid microcarcinomas, recurrences of well-differentiated thyroid carcinoma, and palliation of larger recurrences or poorly differentiated carcinoma have been conducted internationally and have shown promising outcomes of both treatment efficacy and a high level of safety.[40–56] In North America, the role of and appetite for RFA remains undefined for malignant tumors.

Primary malignancy

Growing international evidence suggests the treatment of small papillary thyroid carcinoma (PTC) with RFA may be an effective option in patients who would be candidates for active surveillance or who decline surgery. As of this writing, no major studies have been performed in North America. Several international cohort studies of carefully selected primary papillary thyroid microcarcinomas (PTMC) 10 mm or lesser treated with RFA found near total or total resorption of tumors at 12 months. Core needle biopsy at 3 months posttreatment in one of the studies showed no malignant pathologic condition, and there were no recurrent nodules or cervical lymph node metastases.[42,47] These studies were included in a meta-analysis of 715 patients with PTMC, which found pooled estimates of mean volume reduction of 99.3% for RFA [95% CI 96.2%–102.3%] but a complete disappearance rate of only 65.2% [95% CI 24.3%–100%].[57] Recurrence rate across thermal ablation techniques was 0.4% [95% CI: 0%–1.1%], with mean follow-ups of 7.8 to 25.7 months.

Longer follow-up periods are important in establishing efficacy for malignancy. At a mean follow-up of 42 months (minimum 24 months), Yan and colleagues demonstrated an 88.4% disappearance rate and a malignant progression rate of 3.62% in a large series of 414 patients with PTMC.[58] A 5-year comparison of low-risk PTMC treated with RFA versus surgery demonstrated similar oncologic effectiveness with no significant difference found in recurrent lesions or clinical lymph node metastases, despite 66.3% of the surgeries including a central neck dissection.[48]

Although the subject of active debate and investigation, RFA is currently permissible for primary treatment of very small well-differentiated carcinomas under most society guidelines (surgery remains the recommendation).[8,12,13] Patients are offered surgery, active surveillance, and RFA if appropriate (see **Fig. 1**), and a treatment plan is reached via a shared decision-making model, including consultation with the patient's endocrinologist to ensure long-term follow-up will be available. We emphasize that indefinite follow-up is necessary even if the nodule sonographically resolves, similar to the active surveillance protocol. The Thyroid Cancer-Specific Health-Related Quality of Life Questionnaire is a cancer-specific tool to follow patient symptom burden. Surveillance sonogram interval is poorly defined; our practice is to follow with a repeat ultrasound of the thyroid and cervical lymph nodes at 3, 6, 9, 12, 18, and 24 months for malignant nodules and afterward per endocrinologist surveillance protocol.[8,12,13]

It is tempting to conclude that sonographic resolution is the equivalent of surgical excision of a cancer but we do not have sufficient evidence to make that conclusion. Remnant nodules and ablated parenchyma have the potential to harbor persistent malignancy. Both Ma and colleagues and Sun and colleagues followed patients with thyroid cancers previously treated with RFA but who had suspicious appearance of postablation lesions on ultrasound or new lymph node metastases.[59,60] Persistent malignancy was found in all cases on surgical pathologic condition after thyroidectomy. However, 81% of patients with timeline data available underwent surgery within 60 days of RFA treatment and the volume of treated malignancy at each center was not included, which limits the broader applicability of these studies. Other studies have demonstrated that nodule size increases for many patients during the first year of surveillance (partially due to treatment of the periphery) before involuting by approximately 12 months.[58]

Metastatic and inoperable disease
Interestingly, RFA treatment of local recurrences and metastases is somewhat less controversial. Treatment candidacy is highly variable based on tumor biology, location, size, and earlier treatment as well as patient functional status and comorbidities, and goals of care. Guidelines suggest that patients with limited small cervical recurrences may be treated with curative intent.[13,61] Otherwise, the goal of RFA treatment should be to reduce tumor burden and avoid a potentially morbid surgery that is unlikely to be curative. Extreme caution should be used before treating central neck lesions with RFA, however. The recurrent laryngeal nerve is likely to be adjacent to any tumor recurrence—the benefit from treatment should be carefully weighed against remaining nerve function. In our practice, traditional surgical approaches remain the gold standard for most patients.

Despite these concerns, small recurrences of well-differentiated thyroid cancer may be appropriate for treatment with RFA.[8,12,13] A meta-analysis of 7 studies of localized recurrent thyroid cancers demonstrated a pooled standard mean difference in tumor volume before and after RFA of 0.77 (95% CI 0.57–0.97, reported as proportion of volume reduction not percentage), as well as decrease in thyroglobulin (0.52, 95% CI 0.30–0.73).[62] In a study of small, low-volume PTC recurrences treated with RFA or reoperation, Kim and colleagues found recurrence rates of 11.5% for patients treated with RFA versus 8.7% for patients treated with surgery, with no difference in 1 and 3 year disease-free survival.[63] Choi and colleagues also found no difference in 3 and 6-year recurrence-free survival or serum thyroglobulin levels between RFA and repeat surgery but found a significantly lower rate of initial major complications (voice change >1 month and permanent hypocalcemia) in the RFA group (3.1%) compared with the surgery group (31.2%).[52] Other studies have demonstrated symptom benefit and safety of palliative roles for RFA in debulking tumors that have invaded critical structures (eg, the trachea), other inoperable disease, or in anaplastic thyroid carcinoma.[40,53,54]

Current Controversies/Areas of Further Investigation

Indeterminate nodules
One significant drawback of RFA is the inability to obtain a definitive tissue sample in the case of indeterminate nodules (Bethesda III or IV cytology). The most recent American Head and Neck Society and international guidelines suggest that RFA be avoided in cases of indeterminate nodules. If RFA treatment is to be pursued, it seems prudent to treat all indeterminate nodules as malignant and follow these patients with the same degree of surveillance as patients with cancer diagnoses (see **Fig. 1**).[8,12,13] We do not override cytology (ie, we do not consider "benign" molecular testing to be equivalent to benign FNAB results) but find molecular markers to be informative in patient counseling.

"Doing less" for small, well-differentiated thyroid cancer
The 2015 revised guidelines of the American Thyroid Association for the treatment of thyroid nodules and differentiated cancer in 2015 allowed for active surveillance of very low-risk patients with papillary thyroid microcarcinomas.[64,65] Adoption of active surveillance has been limited however, despite qualitative studies demonstrating patient preferences for more minimally invasive treatment or avoiding surgery.[66,67] If demonstrated to be noninferior to surgery in the long-term, RFA may ultimately serve as the "Goldilocks" treatment between active surveillance and surgery for many patients with small, well-differentiated thyroid cancer that balances the overall excellent prognosis for thyroid cancer with postprocedural quality of life.

High out-of-pocket costs

In addition to its multitude of patient benefits, RFA also carries a substantial opportunity to improve health system expenditures: RFA is estimated to cost 24% to 55% of open thyroid surgery, with largest drivers in cost being facility overhead and the RF electrode.[68–70] However, there is no separate current procedural terminology (CPT) code for RFA (it is an "unlisted procedure, endocrine system"), and inconsistent and inadequate insurance reimbursement often makes the procedure otherwise cost-prohibitive for the performing facility. In the United States, the procedure is typically paid out of pocket by the patient, with estimates ranging from US$5000 to US$9000.[69,71] Although this cost is very high relative to the insurance copays associated with thyroid surgery, it is comparable to other elective (but quality of life improving) medical procedures such as laser refractive eye surgery, which typically ranges from US$4000 to US$6000 for treatment of 2 eyes.[72–74]

SUMMARY

Although RFA of BTNs is relatively new in North America, RFA has an established international record of achieving significant volume reduction for benign nodules in most patients when performed by experienced providers. This minimally invasive technique can be performed in an outpatient or clinic setting, and offers the ability to improve compressive and cosmetic symptoms from thyroid nodules with minimal down time and a low complication rate. Surgery remains the recommendation for thyroid cancer and autonomous functioning nodules in most circumstances, although RFA may offer an alternative to active surveillance for very low-risk cancers. Further investigation is required to elucidate the long-term efficacy of RFA, understand radiologic properties of treated nodules, and investigate the role of RFA for malignant and indeterminate nodules in the North American population.

CLINICS CARE POINTS

- RFA is a minimally invasive procedure performed under ultrasound guidance with an established international record of achieving volume reduction for BTNs in most patients, with an excellent safety profile when performed by experienced providers.
- Nodule volume reduction after RFA correlates with improved compressive and cosmetic symptoms from BTNs.
- Surgery remains the standard of care for initial treatment of thyroid cancer and hyperthyroidism; further investigation in these areas is needed.
- RFA is an alternative to surgery for curative treatment of very limited cervical thyroid cancer recurrences or palliative treatment of bulkier disease and may have a role as an alternative to active surveillance for patients with small, well-differentiated thyroid cancer.

DISCLOSURE

Dr J.O. Russell receives funding from a National Institutes of Health, United States R44 SBIR grant, is currently a site principal investigator for a clinical trial with Eli Lilly, and consults for Baxter International, Inc. Dr K.M. Frazier has no disclosures.

REFERENCES

1. Welbourn RB. Highlights from endocrine surgical history. World J Surg 1996; 20(5). https://doi.org/10.1007/s002689900093.

2. Slough CM, Liddy W, Brooks J, et al. History of thyroid and parathyroid surgery. In: Randolph GW, editor. *Surgery of the thyroid and parathyroid glands.* 3rd edition. Philadelphia, PA: Elsevier; 2021. p. 2–14.

3. Dupuy DE, Monchik JM, Decrea C, et al. Radiofrequency ablation of regional recurrence from well-differentiated thyroid malignancy. Surgery 2001;130(6). https://doi.org/10.1067/msy.2001.118708.

4. Kim YS, Rhim H, Tae K, et al. Techniques in thyroidology radiofrequency ablation of benign cold thyroid nodules: initial clinical experience. Thyroid 2006;16(4): 361–7. www.liebertpub.com.

5. Spiezia S, Garberoglio R, Di Somma C, et al. Efficacy and safety of radiofrequency thermal ablation in the treatment of thyroid nodules with pressure symptoms in elderly patients [5]. J Am Geriatr Soc 2007;55(9):1478–9.

6. Jeong WK, Baek JH, Rhim H, et al. Radiofrequency ablation of benign thyroid nodules: Safety and imaging follow-up in 236 patients. Eur Radiol 2008;18(6). https://doi.org/10.1007/s00330-008-0880-6.

7. Na DG, Lee JH, Jung SL, et al. Radiofrequency ablation of benign Thyroid nodules and recurrent Thyroid cancers: Consensus statement and recommendations. Korean J Radiol 2012;13(2). https://doi.org/10.3348/kjr.2012.13.2.117.

8. Kim JH, Baek JH, Lim HK, et al. 2017 Thyroid radiofrequency ablation guideline: Korean society of thyroid radiology. Korean J Radiol 2018;19(4). https://doi.org/10.3348/kjr.2018.19.4.632.

9. Deandrea M, Sung JY, Limone P, et al. Efficacy and safety of radiofrequency ablation versus observation for nonfunctioning benign thyroid nodules: a randomized controlled international collaborative trial. Thyroid 2015;25(8). https://doi.org/10.1089/thy.2015.0133.

10. Hamidi O, Callstrom MR, Lee RA, et al. Outcomes of radiofrequency ablation therapy for large benign thyroid nodules: a mayo clinic case series. Mayo Clin Proc 2018;93(8). https://doi.org/10.1016/j.mayocp.2017.12.011.

11. Papini E, Monpeyssen H, Frasoldati A, et al. . 2020 European thyroid association clinical practice guideline for the use of image-guided ablation in benign thyroid nodules. Eur Thyroid J 2020;9(4):172–85.

12. Mauri G, Hegedüs L, Bandula S, et al. european thyroid association and cardiovascular and interventional radiological society of europe 2021 clinical practice guideline for the use of minimally invasive treatments in malignant thyroid lesions. Eur Thyroid J 2021;10(3). https://doi.org/10.1159/000516469.

13. Orloff LA, Noel JE, Stack BC, et al. Radiofrequency ablation and related ultrasound-guided ablation technologies for treatment of benign and malignant thyroid disease: An international multidisciplinary consensus statement of the American Head and Neck Society Endocrine Surgery Section with the Asia Pacific Society of Thyroid Surgery, Associazione Medici Endocrinologi, British Association of Endocrine and Thyroid Surgeons, European Thyroid Association, Italian Society of Endocrine Surgery Units, Korean Society of Thyroid. Head Neck 2022; 44(3):633–60.

14. Goldberg SN. Radiofrequency tumor ablation: Principles and techniques. Eur J Ultrasound 2001;13(2). https://doi.org/10.1016/S0929-8266(01)00126-4.

15. Baek JH, Lee JH, Valcavi R, et al. Thermal ablation for benign thyroid nodules: Radiofrequency and laser. Korean J Radiol 2011;12(5):525–40.

16. Lee MK, Baek JH, Suh CH, et al. Clinical practice guidelines for radiofrequency ablation of benign thyroid nodules: A systematic review. Ultrasonography 2021; 40(2). https://doi.org/10.14366/usg.20015.

17. Ben Hamou A, Ghanassia E, Muller A, et al. SFE-AFCE-SFMN 2022 consensus on the management of thyroid nodules: Thermal ablation. Ann Endocrinol 2022; 83(6). https://doi.org/10.1016/j.ando.2022.10.011.

18. Kandil E, Issa PP, Randolph GW. Can Thyroid Nodules be Managed with Radiofrequency Ablation? Adv Surg 2023. https://doi.org/10.1016/j.yasu.2023.05.004.

19. Wolff S, Gałązka A, Dedecjus M. Transcutaneous laryngeal ultrasonography in vocal fold assessment before and after thyroid surgery in light of recent studies. Pol J Radiol 2022;87(1). https://doi.org/10.5114/pjr.2022.115154.

20. Shin JH, Baek JH, Ha EJ, et al. Radiofrequency ablation of thyroid nodules: Basic principles and clinical application. Int J Endocrinol 2012;2012. https://doi.org/10.1155/2012/919650.

21. Tufano RP, Pace-Asciak P, Russell JO, et al. Update of Radiofrequency Ablation for Treating Benign and Malignant Thyroid Nodules. The Future Is Now. Front Endocrinol 2021;12. https://doi.org/10.3389/fendo.2021.698689.

22. Laeseke PF, Sampson LA, Brace CL, et al. Unintended thermal injuries from radiofrequency ablation: Protection with 5% dextrose in water. Am J Roentgenol 2006;186(5 SUPPL). https://doi.org/10.2214/AJR.04.1240.

23. Deandrea M, Trimboli P, Mormile A, et al. Determining an energy threshold for optimal volume reduction of benign thyroid nodules treated by radiofrequency ablation. Eur Radiol 2021;31(7). https://doi.org/10.1007/s00330-020-07532-y.

24. Deandrea M, Trimboli P, Garino F, et al. Long-Term Efficacy of a Single Session of RFA for Benign Thyroid Nodules: A Longitudinal 5-Year Observational Study. J Clin Endocrinol Metab 2019;104(9). https://doi.org/10.1210/jc.2018-02808.

25. Lim HK, Lee JH, Ha EJ, et al. Radiofrequency ablation of benign non-functioning thyroid nodules: 4-year follow-up results for 111 patients. Eur Radiol 2013;23(4). https://doi.org/10.1007/s00330-012-2671-3.

26. Muhammad H, Santhanam P, Russell JO. Radiofrequency ablation and thyroid nodules: updated systematic review. Endocrine 2021;72(3). https://doi.org/10.1007/s12020-020-02598-6.

27. Cho SJ, Baek JH, Chung SR, et al. Long-term results of thermal ablation of benign thyroid nodules: A systematic review and meta-analysis. Endocrinology and Metabolism 2020;35(2). https://doi.org/10.3803/EnM.2020.35.2.339.

28. Spiezia S, Garberoglio R, Milone F, et al. Thyroid nodules and related symptoms are stably controlled two years after radiofrequency thermal ablation. Thyroid 2009;19(3). https://doi.org/10.1089/thy.2008.0202.

29. National Guideline Centre (UK). Management of non-malignant thyroid Enlargement: thyroid disease: assessment and management. London: National Institute for Health and Care Excellence (NICE); 2019.

30. Kandil E, Omar M, Aboueisha M, et al. Efficacy and Safety of Radiofrequency Ablation of Thyroid Nodules: A Multi-institutional Prospective Cohort Study. Ann Surg 2022;276(4). https://doi.org/10.1097/SLA.0000000000005594.

31. Sim JS, Baek JH. Long-term outcomes following thermal ablation of benign thyroid nodules as an alternative to surgery: The importance of controlling regrowth. Endocrinology and Metabolism 2019;34(2). https://doi.org/10.3803/EnM.2019.34.2.117.

32. Li Y, Li W, Jiang B, et al. Analysis and prediction of regrowth in benign thyroid nodules undergoing radiofrequency ablation: a retrospective study with a 5-year follow-up. Eur Radiol 2023. https://doi.org/10.1007/s00330-023-09481-8.

33. Deandrea M, Garino F, Alberto M, et al. Radiofrequency ablation for benign thyroid nodules according to different ultrasound features: An Italian multicentre

prospective study. Eur J Endocrinol 2019;180(1). https://doi.org/10.1530/EJE-18-0685.

34. Wu MH, Chen KY, Chen A, et al. Differences in the ultrasonographic appearance of thyroid nodules after radiofrequency ablation. Clin Endocrinol 2021;95(3). https://doi.org/10.1111/cen.14480.

35. Chung SR, Baek JH, Suh CH, et al. Safety of Radiofrequency Ablation of Benign Thyroid Nodules and Recurrent Thyroid Cancers: A Systematic Review and Meta-Analysis. Ultrasound Med Biol 2017;43. https://doi.org/10.1016/j.ultrasmedbio. 2017.08.1833.

36. Wang JF, Wu T, Hu KP, et al. Complications following radiofrequency ablation of benign thyroid nodules: A systematic review. Chin Med J 2017;130(11). https://doi.org/10.4103/0366-6999.206347.

37. Cesareo R, Palermo A, Pasqualini V, et al. Radiofrequency Ablation on Autonomously Functioning Thyroid Nodules: A Critical Appraisal and Review of the Literature. Front Endocrinol 2020;11. https://doi.org/10.3389/fendo.2020.00317.

38. Cesareo R, Naciu AM, Iozzino M, et al. Nodule size as predictive factor of efficacy of radiofrequency ablation in treating autonomously functioning thyroid nodules. Int J Hyperther 2018;34(5). https://doi.org/10.1080/02656736.2018.1430868.

39. Dobnig H, Amrein K. Monopolar Radiofrequency Ablation of Thyroid Nodules: A Prospective Austrian Single-Center Study. Thyroid 2018;28(4). https://doi.org/10. 1089/thy.2017.0547.

40. Jeong SY, Baek JH, Choi YJ, et al. Radiofrequency ablation of primary thyroid carcinoma: efficacy according to the types of thyroid carcinoma. Int J Hyperther 2018;34(5). https://doi.org/10.1080/02656736.2018.1427288.

41. Kim JH, Baek JH, Sung JY, et al. Radiofrequency ablation of low-risk small papillary thyroidcarcinoma: preliminary results for patients ineligible for surgery. Int J Hyperther 2017;33(2). https://doi.org/10.1080/02656736.2016.1230893.

42. Zhang M, Luo Y, Zhang Y, et al. Efficacy and safety of ultrasound-guided radiofrequency ablation for treating low-risk papillary thyroid microcarcinoma: A prospective study. Thyroid 2016;26(11). https://doi.org/10.1089/thy.2015.0471.

43. Zhu Y, Che Y, Gao S, et al. Long-term follow-up results of PTMC treated by ultrasound-guided radiofrequency ablation: a retrospective study. Int J Hyperther 2021;38(1). https://doi.org/10.1080/02656736.2021.1963850.

44. Tong M, Li S, Li Y, et al. Efficacy and safety of radiofrequency, microwave and laser ablation for treating papillary thyroid microcarcinoma: a systematic review and meta-analysis. Int J Hyperther 2019;36(1). https://doi.org/10.1080/02656736. 2019.1700559.

45. Kim HJ, Cho SJ, Baek JH. Comparison of thermal ablation and surgery for low-risk papillary thyroid microcarcinoma: A systematic review and meta-analysis. Korean J Radiol 2021;22(10). https://doi.org/10.3348/KJR.2020.1308.

46. Lim HK, Cho SJ, Baek JH, et al. US-guided radiofrequency ablation for low-risk papillary thyroid microcarcinoma: Efficacy and safety in a large population. Korean J Radiol 2019;20(12). https://doi.org/10.3348/kjr.2019.0192.

47. Ding M, Tang X, Cui D, et al. Clinical outcomes of ultrasound-guided radiofrequency ablation for the treatment of primary papillary thyroid microcarcinoma. Clin Radiol 2019;74(9). https://doi.org/10.1016/j.crad.2019.05.012.

48. Zhang M, Tufano RP, Russell JO, et al. Ultrasound-Guided Radiofrequency Ablation Versus Surgery for Low-Risk Papillary Thyroid Microcarcinoma: Results of over 5 Years' Follow-Up. Thyroid 2020;30(3). https://doi.org/10.1089/thy.2019.0147.

49. Ito Y, Miyauchi A, Oda H. Low-risk papillary microcarcinoma of the thyroid: A review of active surveillance trials. Eur J Surg Oncol 2018;44(3). https://doi.org/10.1016/j.ejso.2017.03.004.

50. Chung SR, Baek JH, Choi YJ, et al. Longer-term outcomes of radiofrequency ablation for locally recurrent papillary thyroid cancer. Eur Radiol 2019;29(9). https://doi.org/10.1007/s00330-019-06063-5.

51. Suh CH, Baek JH, Choi YJ, et al. Efficacy and safety of radiofrequency and ethanol ablation for treating locally recurrent thyroid cancer: A systematic review and meta-analysis. Thyroid 2016;26(3). https://doi.org/10.1089/thy.2015.0545.

52. Choi Y, Jung SL, Bae JS, et al. Comparison of efficacy and complications between radiofrequency ablation and repeat surgery in the treatment of locally recurrent thyroid cancers: a single-center propensity score matching study. Int J Hyperther 2019;36(1). https://doi.org/10.1080/02656736.2019.1571248.

53. Chung SR, Baek JH, Choi YJ, et al. Efficacy of radiofrequency ablation for recurrent thyroid cancer invading the airways. Eur Radiol 2021;31(4). https://doi.org/10.1007/s00330-020-07283-w.

54. Park KW, Shin JH, Han BK, et al. Inoperable symptomatic recurrent thyroid cancers: Preliminary result of radiofrequency ablation. Ann Surg Oncol 2011;18(9). https://doi.org/10.1245/s10434-011-1619-1.

55. Chen WC, Chou CK, Chang YH, et al. Efficacy of radiofrequency ablation for metastatic papillary thyroid cancer with and without initial biochemical complete status. Front Endocrinol 2022;13. https://doi.org/10.3389/fendo.2022.933931.

56. Lee SJ, Jung SL, Kim BS, et al. Radiofrequency ablation to treat loco-regional recurrence of well-differentiated thyroid carcinoma. Korean J Radiol 2014;15(6). https://doi.org/10.3348/kjr.2014.15.6.817.

57. Choi Y, Jung SL. Efficacy and Safety of Thermal Ablation Techniques for the Treatment of Primary Papillary Thyroid Microcarcinoma: A Systematic Review and Meta-Analysis. Thyroid 2020;30(5). https://doi.org/10.1089/thy.2019.0707.

58. Yan L, Lan Y, Xiao J, et al. Long-term outcomes of radiofrequency ablation for unifocal low-risk papillary thyroid microcarcinoma: a large cohort study of 414 patients. Eur Radiol 2021;31(2). https://doi.org/10.1007/s00330-020-07128-6.

59. Sun W, Zhang H, He L, et al. Surgery after ultrasound-guided radiofrequency ablation for papillary thyroid carcinoma in 21 patients: A retrospective study from a single center in China. Med Sci Mon Int Med J Exp Clin Res 2020;26. https://doi.org/10.12659/MSM.928391.

60. Ma B, Wei W, Xu W, et al. Surgical Confirmation of Incomplete Treatment for Primary Papillary Thyroid Carcinoma by Percutaneous Thermal Ablation: A Retrospective Case Review and Literature Review. Thyroid 2018;28(9). https://doi.org/10.1089/thy.2017.0558.

61. Jeong SY, Baek JH, Choi YJ, et al. Ethanol and thermal ablation for malignant thyroid tumours. Int J Hyperther 2017;33(8). https://doi.org/10.1080/02656736.2017.1361048.

62. Zhao Q, Tian G, Kong D, et al. Meta-analysis of radiofrequency ablation for treating the local recurrence of thyroid cancers. J Endocrinol Invest 2016;39(8). https://doi.org/10.1007/s40618-016-0450-8.

63. Kim JH, Yoo WS, Park YJ, et al. Efficacy and safety of radiofrequency ablation for treatment of locally recurrent thyroid cancers smaller than 2 cm. Radiology 2015;276(3). https://doi.org/10.1148/radiol.15140079.

64. Haugen BR, Alexander EK, Bible KC, et al. 2015 American thyroid association management guidelines for adult patients with thyroid nodules and differentiated

thyroid cancer: the american thyroid association guidelines task force on thyroid nodules and differentiated thyroid cancer. Thyroid 2016;26(1):1–133.

65. Haugen BR. 2015 American Thyroid Association Management Guidelines for Adult Patients with Thyroid Nodules and Differentiated Thyroid Cancer: What is new and what has changed? Cancer 2017;123(3). https://doi.org/10.1002/cncr.30360.

66. Kim J, Roth EG, Carlisle K, et al. Eliciting Low-Risk Thyroid Cancer Treatment Preferences Using Clinical Vignettes: A Pilot Study. Endocr Pract 2023;29(7). https://doi.org/10.1016/j.eprac.2023.04.008.

67. Pace-Asciak P, Russell JO, Tufano RP. Review: Improving quality of life in patients with differentiated thyroid cancer. Front Oncol 2023;13. https://doi.org/10.3389/fonc.2023.1032581.

68. Schalch MS, Costa ACN, de Souza RP, et al. Radiofrequency ablation of thyroid nodules: prospective cost-effectiveness analysis in comparison to conventional thyroidectomy. Arch Endocrinol Metab 2021;65(6). https://doi.org/10.20945/2359-3997000000411.

69. Kuo EJ, Oh A, Hu Y, et al. If the price is right: Cost-effectiveness of radiofrequency ablation versus thyroidectomy in the treatment of benign thyroid nodules. Surgery (United States) 2023;173. https://doi.org/10.1016/j.surg.2022.08.048.

70. Miller JR, Tanavde V, Razavi C, et al. Cost comparison between open thyroid lobectomy and radiofrequency ablation for management of thyroid nodules. Head Neck 2023;45(1). https://doi.org/10.1002/hed.27213.

71. Ayoub NF, Balakrishnan K, Orloff LA, et al. Time-driven Activity-based cost comparison of thyroid Lobectomy and radiofrequency ablation. Otolaryngol Head Neck Surg; 2023. https://doi.org/10.1002/ohn.360.

72. Camejo MD, Rupani MK, Rebenitsch RL. A comparative analysis of the cost of cataract surgery abroad and in the United States. Indian J Ophthalmol 2014;62(6). https://doi.org/10.4103/0301-4738.136288.

73. Agyekum S, Chan PP, Zhang Y, et al. Cost-effectiveness analysis of myopia management: A systematic review. Front Public Health 2023;11. https://doi.org/10.3389/fpubh.2023.1093836.

74. Patil SA, Luu A, Vail DG, et al. Utilization of Crowdfunding for Cataract and LASIK Procedures. Semin Ophthalmol 2022;37(5). https://doi.org/10.1080/08820538.2022.2054664.

Secondary Hyperparathyroidism

Brendan C. Stack Jr, MD

KEYWORDS

- Secondary hyperparathyroidism • Dialysis • Chronic kidney disease • Parathyroid

KEY POINTS

- Secondary hyperparathyroidism (SHPT) is a manifestation of a chronic condition that classically occurs from chronic kidney disease.
- SHPT is largely managed through diet, ultraviolet exposure, vitamin D intake, and dialysis.
- SHPT may require surgery in cases of severe electrolyt imbalance or in preparatation for kidney transplant.

PARATHYROID PHYSIOLOGY

There is equilibrium in parathyroid physiology between calcium and parathyroid hormone (PTH). It is helpful to think of these 2 elements on a balance, when one decreases, the other increases. The physiologic response is for the PTH to rise when calcium is lowered and vice versa. Parathyroid changes are affected by the glands themselves mediated by their calcium-sensing receptors (CaSR). Calcium is regulated In circulation through 2 broad mechanisms: calcium in circulation or sequestration. Forces to correct hypocalcemia includes renal retention, intestinal absorption, and skeletal matrix breakdown. Sequestration of calcium in an effort to address hypercalcemia includes urinary excretion, intestinal exclusion, and skeletal deposition of calcium (**Fig. 1**).[1]

EPIDEMIOLOGY OF SECONDARY HYPERPARATHYROIDISM

SHPT is most commonly associated with vitamin D deficiency or chronic kidney disease (CKD).[1] Severe vitamin D deficiency (<30 nmol/L [<12 ng/mL]) is seen in approximately 7%.[1–5] US National Health and Nutrition Examination Survey (https://www.cdc.gov/nchs/nhanes/index) of 2010 data estimate that the prevalence of 25-hydroxyvitamin D levels of less than 30 nmol/L (<12 ng/mL) is 6.7% in the US population.[6] Vitamin D deficiency is a more significant contributor to SHPT in developed societies.

Department of Otolaryngology-HNS Southern Illinois University/SIU Medicine, 720 North Bond Street, PO Box 19662, Springfield, IL 62794-9662, USA
E-mail address: bcstackjr@gmail.com

Otolaryngol Clin N Am 57 (2024) 99–110
https://doi.org/10.1016/j.otc.2023.07.010
0030-6665/24/© 2023 Elsevier Inc. All rights reserved.

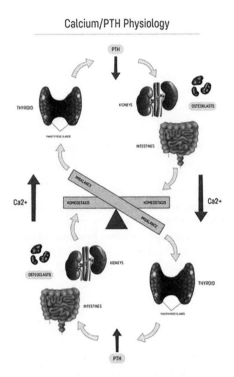

Fig. 1. The physiologic balance of calcium and parathyroid hormone. Upper and lower loops demonstrate the correction for elevated and reduced calcium, respectively. The calcium-sensing receptors of the parathyroid manage calcium physiology.

The estimated global prevalence of all-stage CKD in 2017 was 9%.[7] Over 80% of patients with CKD are at risk for the development of vitamin D deficiency, with an inverse correlation between decreasing 25-hydroxyvitamin D levels and elevated PTH across all stages of CKD.[8] Elevation of PTH levels begins around a glomerular filtration rate (GFR) of 45 mL/min/1.73 m^2 and increases as GFR levels decline.[9–13]

The incidence of parathyroidectomy in patients with chronic renal failure has declined to 5.28 per 1000 patient years.[14–16] This reduction may be related to improved medical treatment in the early stages of renal disease. The prevalence of SHPT caused by vitamin D deficiency was noted to be 30.2% in a study from Boston in patients over 65 living in low-income housing.[17,18] The incidence was greater among African American elderly than among whites.

PATHOPHYSIOLOGY OF SECONDARY HYPERPARATHYROIDISM

PTH is released by the parathyroids and maintains calcium homeostasis by acting on the renal tubules, on calcium stores in the skeleton, and indirectly on the gastrointestinal tract through both activation of vitamin D and enteral calcium absorption (see **Fig. 1**). SHPT most commonly occurs in the setting of decreased levels of 1,25-dihydroxy vitamin D, hyperphosphatemia, and hypocalcemia.[19] Phosphorus levels begin to climb once the GFR decreases below 20 cm^3/min and serves as another stimulus for PTH.

Chronic Kidney Disease

Signs and symptoms of advanced CKD include skin discoloration, bruising, pruritus, lung rales, pericardial rub, edema, fatigue, nausea, poor concentration or memory, and myoclonus.[20,21] SHPT symptoms such as arthritis, bone pain, myopathy, tendon rupture, and extraskeletal calcifications are common; however, with advances in medical therapy and earlier intervention, patients with SHPT are usually asymptomatic.[22] Imaging for vascular or cardiac valvular calcification should be considered because patients with CKD–mineral bone disorder (MBD) have a high cardiovascular risk.[2]

In CKD, there is a loss of 1-alpha-hydroxylase in the kidney which decreases the conversion of 25-hydroxy vitamin D into the active 1,25-dihydroxy form. Low levels of 1,25-dihydroxy vitamin D, with or without hypocalcemia, are detected by CaSR and results in increased PTH. Fat malabsorption that binds dietary vitamin D enterally and contributes to reduced absorption of vitamin D (fat soluble) and dietary calcium (compounded by inadequate intake) ultimately leads to hypocalcemia and increased PTH.[3,22]

Resected parathyroids in SHPT show diffuse and nodular hyperplasia on histology.[19] Hyperplasia has a decreased expression of CaSR, which is thought to increase PTH secretion.[20] Nodular parathyroid tissue has an abnormality in the vitamin D receptor which also increases PTH. The degree of PTH elevation has been correlated with the enlargement of the gland in patients with SHPT.[21–23] Coronary artery calcification and calciphylaxis contribute to a high mortality rate. Both complications have been related to an elevated calcium-phosphorus product.[23,24] Risk factors include length of dialysis, high calcium-phosphorus product, and daily calcium intake.[25] Other causes of SHPT resulting from low levels of vitamin D are chronic illness, liver disease, or medications that increase the clearance of 25-hydroxyvitamin D or impair the 25-hydroxylation (**Box 1**).

Vitamin D

Exposure to sunlight is the major source of vitamin D.[3] There are 2 main forms of vitamin D: colecalciferol (vitamin D3, animal derived) and ergocalciferol (vitamin D2, plant derived). Ergocalciferol (vitamin D2) has a different side chain from colecalciferol. Colecalciferol occurs in relatively few foods: salmon, tuna, mackerel, and fish-liver oils, with smaller amounts found in beef liver, cheese, and egg yolks.[26]

Once vitamin D is made in the skin or ingested, it undergoes 2 hydroxylations, the first in the liver to form 25-hydroxy vitamin D. This compound, bound to vitamin D-binding protein (DBP), travels to the kidney where the megalin receptor translocates the DBP–25-hydroxy vitamin D complex into the renal tubule. The enzyme 25-hydroxy

---

Box 1
Differential of etiologies of secondary hyperparathyroidism

- Diminished intake of calcium

- Calcium loss
  - After pregnancy and breastfeeding
  - Bisphosphonate treatment
  - Idiopathic hypercalciuria
  - Loop diuretics
  - Rhabdomyolysis
  - Sepsis

- Diminished parathormone effect

- Pseudohypoparathyroidism (G-protein deficiency).

vitamin D-1-alpha-hydroxylase (CYP27 B) introduces a hydroxyl group to form 1,25-dihydroxy vitamin D.[3] Fibroblast growth factor-23 is an important regulator of vitamin D metabolism.[27,28] Chronic vitamin D deficiency results in osteomalacia and decreased bone densities.[13]

In the intestines, 1,25-dihydroxy vitamin D induces the expression of an epithelial calcium channel, calcium-binding protein (calbindin), and other proteins that transport calcium from the diet into circulation.[3] 1,25-Dihydroxy vitamin D also interacts with nuclear vitamin D receptors in osteoblasts to stimulate the expression of the receptor activator of nuclear factor kappa-B ligand (RANKL), which leads to osteoclast maturation and bone resorption. The RANKL protein is recognized by the receptor activator of nuclear factor kappa-B (RANK) present on the plasma membrane of preosteoclasts, and the RANKL–RANK interaction results in the increase and maturation of osteoclasts.[22,29]

PTH acts to increase ionized calcium by interacting with membrane receptors on mature osteoblasts, which induces the expression of RANKL. PTH also decreases the gene expression of osteoprotegerin (a decoy receptor for RANKL) in osteoblasts, which enhances osteoclastogenesis. The osteoclasts release hydrochloric acid and collagenases to disintegrate bone resulting in the mobilization of calcium.[22]

Another effect of vitamin D deficiency is the loss of phosphorus in the urine.[29] The inadequate calcium–phosphorus product that results causes the bone matrix to be poorly mineralized. In children, the weight of the body causes the skeleton to develop classical rachitic deformities such as bowed legs or knocked knees. In adults, there is generally sufficient skeletal mineralization to prevent skeletal deformities, although in a vitamin D-deficient state newly laid-down osteoid cannot be properly mineralized, leading to osteomalacia.[19] This is associated with throbbing bone pain (commonly affecting the pelvis, hips, legs (shins), lower back, or ribs), often misdiagnosed as fibromyalgia, myositis, or chronic fatigue syndrome.[29]

Sunlight (Ultraviolet B)

Exposure to sunlight is the major source of vitamin D.[3] Concerns of increased skin cancers (melanoma) due to ultraviolet radiation resulted in successful campaigns to minimize sun exposure during the precise time of day, vitamin D is best synthesized.[27] Inadequate vitamin D exposure is common among older patients, particularly those who always use sunblock, are housebound or institutionalized.[28] If inadequate sun exposure is identified as a factor in vitamin D insufficiency and SHPT, advice on safe sun exposure should be explained. Exposure to sunlight depends on physical factors (eg, latitude, season, weather, time of day) and personal factors (eg, skin pigmentation, body surface area exposed, sun cream use).[3,5,26,29]

Vitamin D-containing dietary supplements may be given. In some countries, many dairy products, juice and juice drinks, and cereals are fortified with vitamin D, and their consumption should be encouraged as part of a balanced diet in people at risk of vitamin D deficiency. Calcium supplements may also be appropriate in conjunction with vitamin D.

Chronic Kidney Disease–Mineral Bone Disorder

SHPT is important in CKD–MBD. CKD–MBD is defined as aberrant mineral and bone metabolism due to CKD manifested by the following: abnormalities of calcium, phosphorus, PTH, or vitamin D metabolism; abnormalities in bone turnover, mineralization, volume, linear growth, or strength; vascular or other soft tissue calcifications.[1,2,6] Parathyroidectomy may be required to remove irreversibly enlarged parathyroid glands. This will be a focus of this study as it is an effective means to mitigate the metabolic ramifications of long-term kidney failure or prepare a patient for renal transplantation.

SECONDARY HYPERPARATHYROIDISM DIAGNOSIS

There is no single test to diagnose SHPT; however, an elevated PTH level with low serum calcium is characteristic. If the phosphorus is elevated, the cause is likely chronic renal failure. If the serum phosphorus is low, then vitamin D deficiency is likely. If vitamin D levels are low, malabsorption syndromes, inadequate sunlight exposure, and other abnormalities should be considered.[22]

Clinical Features

Severe vitamin D deficiency and hypocalcemia present with neuromuscular irritability.[30,31] Hypocalcemia is suggested by Chvostek's sign (tapping on the face just anterior to the ear produces twitching of muscles around the mouth) or Trousseau's sign (inflating a blood-pressure cuff above diastolic for about 3 minutes causes muscular flexion of the wrist, hyperextension of the fingers, and flexion of the thumb). Malabsorption may arise from several conditions.[29]

Laboratory Testing

Laboratory investigations are required to confirm elevated PTH and hypocalcemia and to help establish the underlying cause. Initial investigations should include PTH, calcium, phosphorus, 25-hydroxyvitamin D, and assessment of renal function.[22,32,33] Important labs to include are depicted in **Box 2**.

THERAPY FOR SECONDARY HYPERPARATHYROIDISM

Vitamin D replacement and phosphorus reduction are the mainstays of management. Advances in phosphorus-binding drugs have been helpful in reducing serum phosphorus without raising calcium. Sevelamer is a phosphorus binder that does not contain calcium or aluminum and helps limit calcium absorption. Vitamin D formulations are limited by toxicities including hypercalcemia and hyperphosphatemia. These agents should not be used unless the serum phosphorus is less than 6 mg/dL. Newer vitamin D analogs, paricalcitol, and doxercalciferol may reduce PTH with less toxicity. These analogs are designed to activate the vitamin D receptor selectively at the parathyroid gland while minimizing the calcemic activity typical of vitamin D.[34–36]

Malabsorption

Patients with intestinal malabsorption syndromes are often vitamin D and calcium deficient. The best method to correct vitamin D deficiency is sensible sun exposure.[3] This may be augmented with oral supplements of vitamin D and calcium. Treatment of the underlying intestinal disease should also be optimized.

Vitamin D

The body uses an average of 3000 to 5000 international units (IU) of colecalciferol per day.[37] In the absence of adequate sun exposure, it is estimated that 1000 IU daily of colecalciferol is needed to maintain a healthy 25-hydroxyvitamin D level of at least 75 nmol/L (30 ng/mL).[26] Oral supplementation is most common but intramuscular injection might be used in cases of malabsorption.

Chronic Kidney Disease

PTH levels increase as the GFR declines[1,2,9] (**Box 3**). Serum PTH levels are widely used as indicators for CKD-related SHPT and initiating therapy but may be unreliable.[1,2] Trends in PTH are clinically relevant and useful in guiding treatment. The Kidney Disease: Improving Global Outcomes guidelines recommend that patients with

---

Box 2
Laboratories for secondary hyperparathyroidism

Intact parathyroid hormone (iPTH)
- Elevation of iPTH is the definitive test to establish hyperparathyroidism. iPTH should always be ordered with a paired calcium level so that the iPTH level can be properly interpreted. PTH levels vary over the course of a day, peaking at about 2 AM. Specimens are usually taken at about 8 AM.
  - Stracke S, Keller F, Steinbach G, et al. Long-term outcome after total parathyroidectomy for the management of secondary hyperparathyroidism. Nephron Clin Pract. 2009;111(2):c102 to 9.

Calcium level (total or ionized)
- The relationship between the calcium level and the iPTH level is what distinguishes primary (PHTP) from SHPT. In SHPT, the calcium level is low, which causes an increase in the production of PTH in an attempt to increase calcium levels back into the normal range. Total or ionized calcium can be measured, but it is important to use the same test on every occasion to allow accurate comparisons and trend analysis.

25-hydroxyvitamin D
- Evaluation for possible vitamin D deficiency should form part of the work-up of a patient with suspected SHPT as it is the most common reason for PTH elevation.
  - Silverberg SJ. Vitamin D deficiency and primary hyperparathyroidism. J Bone Miner Res. 2007 Dec;22 suppl 2:V100 to 4.
  - Lips P. Vitamin D deficiency and secondary hyperparathyroidism in the elderly: consequences for bone loss and fractures and therapeutic implications. Endocr Rev. 2001 Aug;22(4):477 to 501.
  - Redman C, Bodenner D, Stack B Jr. Role of vitamin D deficiency in continued hyperparathyroidism following parathyroidectomy. Head Neck. 2009 Sep;31(9):1164 to 7.
- The level of 25-hydroxy vitamin D is the most accurate measure of the amount of vitamin D in the body. Other metabolites may be measured, but these do not reflect the total body stores of this fat-soluble vitamin as accurately as 25-hydroxy vitamin D.
  Thresholds for the definition of vitamin D deficiency for the general population differ between advisory bodies. The normal range may vary between laboratories but is usually 40 to 184 nmol/L (16–74 ng/mL). Many experts hold that any value 75 nmol/L (30 ng/mL) or less demonstrates vitamin D insufficiency. If the PTH is elevated and the 25-hydroxyvitamin D level is low, the latter should be corrected first.
  - Christodoulou M, Aspray TJ, Schoenmakers I. Vitamin D supplementation for patients with chronic kidney disease: a systematic review and meta-analyses of trials investigating the response to supplementation and an overview of guidelines. Calcif Tissue Int. 2021 Aug;109(2):157 to 178.
  - Giustina A, Bouillon R, Binkley N, et al. Controversies in vitamin D: a statement from the Third International Conference. JBMR Plus. 2020 Dec;4(12):e10417.

Renal function (blood urea nitrogen [BUN], creatinine, estimate of glomerular filtration rate [eGFR]) and phosphorus
- Serum creatinine, urea, and calculated glomerular filtration rate (GFR) are used to assess renal function. If elevated, they suggest kidney disease, the most serious cause of SHPT.
  - Stevens LA, Coresh J, Greene T, et al. Assessing kidney function - measured and estimated glomerular filtration rate. N Engl J Med. 2006 Jun 8;354(23):2473 to 83.
- Measuring phosphorus levels allows an appreciation of the severity of kidney disease and may indicate the need for phosphorus reduction therapy. If phosphorus levels are low, other anomalies such as vitamin D deficiency are more likely.
  - Fraser WD. Hyperparathyroidism. Lancet. 2009 Jul 11;374(9684):145 to 58.

Magnesium
- Hypomagnesemia and hypermagnesemia can cause tissue resistance to PTH or reduce PTH production, which in turn causes hypocalcemia. Therefore, PTH can be low, normal, or mildly elevated. CKD may result in either hypomagnesemia or hypermagnesemia.
  - Fiorentini D, Cappadone C, Farruggia G, et al. Magnesium: biochemistry, nutrition, detection, and social impact of diseases linked to its deficiency. Nutrients. 2021 Mar 30;13(4):1136.

○ Rodelo-Haad C, Pendón-Ruiz de Mier MV, Díaz-Tocados JM, et al. The role of disturbed Mg homeostasis in chronic kidney disease comorbidities. Front Cell Dev Biol. 2020 Nov 12;8:543,099.

PTH levels that are progressively rising or persistently above the upper limit of normal be evaluated for modifiable factors including low calcium, high phosphate, and vitamin D deficiency. Treatment should not be based on a single elevated PTH value.[1,2] One post-hoc analysis of the OPTIMA study found that serum phosphorus levels in patients on dialysis with SHPT were better controlled when PTH levels were lowered.[35]

If PTH is above the reference range, serum 25-hydroxy vitamin D should be measured[2,37] and vitamin D supplementation should be initiated.[8,36] Vitamin D therapy should be adjusted in light of serum calcium and phosphorus levels (which should be measured at least every 3 months).[1,2] If the serum phosphorus exceeds the normal range, initiate dietary phosphate restrictions, or if hyperphosphatemia persists but the 25-hydroxy vitamin D is less than 75 nmol/L (<30 ng/mL), oral phosphate binder therapy should be initiated.[2] Therapy for hypocalcemia should be individualized and include calcium salts such as calcium carbonate or calcium acetate orally, or calcium gluconate or calcium chloride parenterally, and/or an oral vitamin D.[2]

Management of Parathyroid Hormone Levels in Advanced Chronic Kidney Disease (Stages 4 to 5)

The use of calcitriol and vitamin D analogs should be reserved for patients with CKD stages 4 to 5 with severe and progressive SHPT.[1,2,37] During therapy with vitamin D or analog, serum levels of calcium, PTH, and phosphorus should be monitored at least every month after initiation of therapy for the first 3 months, then at least every 3 months thereafter. Calcimimetic medications, such as cinacalcet, bind to CaSR and increase their sensitivity to extracellular ionized calcium. This results in decreased PTH, calcium, and phosphate levels. The effect on PTH levels can be seen as quickly as 2 to 4 hours after administration. Calcimimetics serve to reset or shift the PTH–calcium curve to the right. Cinacalcet is reserved for CKD stage 5D, where a vitamin D sterol or analog has inadequately suppressed PTH to within the target range, with or without hypercalcemia. There is anecdotal evidence of a reduction in fractures after starting cinacalcet therapy, but this has not been supported by bone densitometry (DEXA) results.[1,2,25]

Box 3
Stages of chronic kidney disease

- Stage 1: Kidney damage with normal or increased GFR (greater than or equal to 90 mL/min/1.73 m^2)

- Stage 2: Kidney damage with mild decrease in GFR (60–89 mL/min/1.73 m^2)

- Stage 3a: Mild-to-moderate decrease in GFR (45–59 mL/min/1.73 m^2)

- Stage 3b: Moderate-to-severe decrease in GFR (30–44 mL/min/1.73 m^2)

- Stage 4: Severe decrease in GFR (15–29 mL/min/1.73 m^2)

- Stage 5: Kidney failure (GFR <15 mL/min/1.73 m^2 or on dialysis [stage 5D])

D suffix denotes on hemodialysis.

Etelcalcetide is a second-generation, type II calcimimetic. It is a novel D-peptide agonist of CaSR and is approved for SHPT in adult patients with CKD on hemodialysis where treatment with a calcimimetic is indicated but cinacalcet is not tolerable or there is poor compliance. A higher rate of hypocalcemia was observed for etelcalcetide compared with cinacalcet (68.9% vs 59.8%).

Parathyroidectomy

If surgical treatment is considered, the modality of imaging used might includes ultrasound, high-resolution contrast computed tomography, MRI, and 99Tc-sestamibi nuclear medicine scans. These are used for surgical planning and not the diagnosis of SHPT. The use of intravenous contrast material needs to be considered in patients with renal compromise as it might worsen poor renal function. If the patient is anuric or on a kidney transplant list, the adverse effects of contrast administration become moot.

Parathyroidectomy is recommended for severe parathormonemia (PTH above 9 times the upper limit of normal) associated with hypercalcemia and/or hyperphosphatemia that are refractory to medical therapy.[1,2,13] Surgery may be desirable for CKD patients in preparation for renal transplantation. The NIH guidelines for surgery for SHPT (or tertiary hyperparathyroidism) are not available as for primary dysfunction of parathyroid glands. Surgery is reserved for patients with refractory disease who have not responded to medical therapy and have symptoms. Compelling reasons for surgery include a desire to avoid cardiovascular complications (a common cause of death in patients with CKD).

Parathyroidectomy for SHPT is less frequent in the United States than in the rest of the world. Parathyroidectomy rates fell with the introduction of new medical therapies for SHPT. One study concluded that subtotal parathyroidectomy was superior to medical management with cinacalcet in achieving normocalcemia (66% vs 100%) in patients greater than 6 months from the time of transplantation.

Effective surgical therapy for severe SHPT can be accomplished by subtotal parathyroidectomy or total parathyroidectomy with parathyroid tissue auto-transplantation (primarily or secondarily after cryopreservation).[2] In subtotal parathyroidectomy, half of the most normal-appearing gland is left behind with an intact vascular pedicle and demonstrable adequate perfusion (usually marked). For total parathyroidectomy, all 4 glands are excised and a portion of 1 gland (most normal appearing) is auto-transplanted in the sternocleidomastoid muscle in the neck, the brachioradialis muscle in the arm (avoid any dialysis shunt), or subcutaneous chest or abdominal adipose. Patients undergoing surgery have a reduction of long-term death of 28% in all-cause mortality and a 37% decrease in cardiovascular mortality. Benefits of surgery include improvements in anemia and quality of life.

The main drawback of surgery is postoperative hypoparathyroidism and severe hypocalcemia. The risk is greater in total parathyroidectomy with auto-transplantation compared with subtotal parathyroidectomy. These patients often have severely demineralized skeletons and can develop a postoperative "hungry bone" syndrome. In patients who undergo parathyroidectomy, in the 72 hours before parathyroidectomy, administration of a vitamin D or analog may lessen postoperative hypocalcemia.

If the blood levels of calcium fall below normal (ie, <0.9 mmol/L [<3.6 mg/dL] ionized calcium corresponding to corrected total calcium of 1.8 mmol/L [7.2 mg/dL]), a calcium gluconate infusion should be initiated. The calcium infusion should be gradually reduced when the level of ionized calcium reaches the normal range and remains stable. When oral intake is possible, the patient should receive calcium carbonate as well as calcitriol. If the patient was receiving phosphate binders before surgery, this therapy may need to be discontinued.

> **Box 4**
> **SHPT-related guidelines**
>
> - Evaluation, treatment, and prevention of vitamin D deficiency, The Endocrine Society, Last published: 2011.
> - Dietary reference intakes for calcium and vitamin D, National Academy of Medicine (Institute of Medicine), Last published: 2011.
> - Chronic kidney disease: assessment and management, National Institute for Health and Care Excellence, Last published: 2021.
> - The European Association of Nuclear Medicine (EANM) practice guidelines for parathyroid imaging, European Association of Nuclear Medicine, Last published: 2021.
> - Assessment criteria for vitamin D deficiency or insufficiency in Japan, The Japan Endocrine Society, Last published: 2017.
> - Kidney Disease: Improving Global Outcomes (KDIGO) clinical practice guideline update for the diagnosis, evaluation, prevention, and treatment of chronic kidney disease–mineral and bone disorder (CKD–MBD), KDIGO, CKD–MBD Work Group, Last published: 2009; selective update 2017.
> - Percutaneous ethanol injection therapy (PEIT), The Japanese Society for Parathyroid Intervention, Last published: 2003.

There is debate around the use of intraoperative adjuncts for the localization of parathyroid glands; there are possible adverse effects associated with methylene blue and fluorescein (near-infrared imaging).[38] Nonsurgical options for parathyroid gland obliteration include thermal (eg, microwave, radiofrequency, laser) and chemical (eg, ethanol) ablation.[39] Calcitriol injection into the parathyroid gland but data are limited.[13] These treatment options are considered in patients who are not candidates for general anesthesia.

SUMMARY

SHPT is largely managed through diet, ultraviolet exposure, vitamin D intake, and dialysis. Drugs and surgery are largely held in reserve for cases of refractory PTH elevation, complications of CKD and comorbid conditions, and in preparation for planned renal transplantation. A team approach to managing these patients is essential. Guidelines are reviewed in **Box 4**.

REFERENCES

1. Khwaja A, Salam S. Secondary Hyperparathyroidism, BMJ Best Practice, Available at: https://bestpractice.bmj.com/topics/en-gb/1107. Accessed May 15, 2023.
2. Ketteler M, Block GA, Evenepoel P, et al. Diagnosis, Evaluation, Prevention, and Treatment of Chronic Kidney Disease-Mineral and Bone Disorder: Synopsis of the Kidney Disease: Improving Global Outcomes 2017 Clinical Practice Guideline Update. Ann Intern Med 2018;168(6):422–30.
3. Holick MF. The vitamin D deficiency pandemic: Approaches for diagnosis, treatment and prevention. Rev Endocr Metab Disord 2017;18(2):153–65.
4. Gong M, Wang K, Sun H, et al. Threshold of 25(OH)D and consequently adjusted parathyroid hormone reference intervals: data mining for relationship between vitamin D and parathyroid hormone. J Endocrinol Invest 2023. https://doi.org/10.1007/s40618-023-02057-9.

5. Giustina A, Bouillon R, Binkley N, et al. Controversies in Vitamin D: A Statement From the Third International Conference. JBMR Plus 2020;4(12):e10417.

6. Schleicher RL, Sternberg MR, Lacher DA, et al. The vitamin D status of the US population from 1988 to 2010 using standardized serum concentrations of 25-hydroxyvitamin D shows recent modest increases. Am J Clin Nutr 2016;104(2): 454–61.

7. GBD Chronic Kidney Disease Collaboration. Global, regional, and national burden of chronic kidney disease, 1990-2017: a systematic analysis for the Global Burden of Disease Study 2017. Lancet 2020;395(10225):709–33.

8. Franca Gois PH, Wolley M, Ranganathan D, et al. Vitamin D Deficiency in Chronic Kidney Disease: Recent Evidence and Controversies. Int J Environ Res Public Health 2018;15(8):1773.

9. Levin A, Bakris GL, Molitch M, et al. Prevalence of abnormal serum vitamin D, PTH, calcium, and phosphorus in patients with chronic kidney disease: results of the study to evaluate early kidney disease. Kidney Int 2007;71(1):31–8.

10. Reddy AC, Nguyen A, McGarvey NH, et al. Factors in nephrologists' decision to treat pre-dialysis CKD patients with vitamin D insufficiency and SHPT: A discrete choice experiment. PLoS One 2023;18(3):e0283531.

11. Min B, Yun SR, Yoon SH, et al. Comparison of the association intensity of creatinine and cystatin C with hyperphosphatemia and hyperparathyroidism in patients with chronic kidney disease. Sci Rep 2023;13(1):3855. PMID: 36890290; PMCID: PMC9995313.

12. Barbuto S, Perrone V, Veronesi C, et al. Real-World Analysis of Outcomes and Economic Burden in Patients with Chronic Kidney Disease with and without Secondary Hyperparathyroidism among a Sample of the Italian Population. Nutrients 2023;15(2):336.

13. Saleem TF, Horwith M, Stack BC Jr. Significance of primary hyperparathyroidism in the management of osteoporosis. Otolaryngol Clin North Am 2004;37(4): 751–61, viii-ix. PMID: 15262513.

14. Ivarsson KM, Akaberi S, Isaksson E, et al. The effect of parathyroidectomy on patient survival in secondary hyperparathyroidism. Nephrol Dial Transplant 2015; 30(12):2027–33.

15. Chen L, Wang K, Yu S, et al. Long-term mortality after parathyroidectomy among chronic kidney disease patients with secondary hyperparathyroidism: a systematic review and meta-analysis. Ren Fail 2016;38(7):1050–8.

16. Miedziaszczyk M, Lacka K, Tomczak O, et al. Systematic Review of the Treatment of Persistent Hyperparathyroidism Following Kidney Transplantation. Biomedicines 2022;11(1):25.

17. Harris SS, Soteriades E, Dawson-Hughes B. Framingham Heart Study; Boston Low-Income Elderly Osteoporosis Study. Secondary hyperparathyroidism and bone turnover in elderly blacks and whites. J Clin Endocrinol Metab 2001;86(8):3801–4.

18. Thomas MK, Lloyd-Jones DM, Thadhani RI, et al. Hypovitaminosis D in medical inpatients. N Engl J Med 1998;338(12):777–83.

19. Ivarsson KM, Akaberi S, Isaksson E, et al. Cardiovascular and Cerebrovascular Events After Parathyroidectomy in Patients on Renal Replacement Therapy. World J Surg 2019;43(8):1981–8.

20. Välimäki S, Farnebo F, Forsberg L, et al. Heterogeneous expression of receptor mRNAs in parathyroid glands of secondary hyperparathyroidism. Kidney Int 2001;60(5):1666–75.

21. Lewin E, Olgaard K. Influence of parathyroid mass on the regulation of PTH secretion. Kidney Int Suppl 2006;(102):S16–21. PMID: 16810305.

22. Fraser WD. Hyperparathyroidism. Lancet 2009;374(9684):145–58.

23. Tominaga Y, Johansson H, Takagi H, et al. Secondary hyperparathyroidism: pathophysiology, histopathology, and medical and surgical management. Surg Today 1997;27(9):787–92.

24. Hutcheson JD, Goettsch C. Cardiovascular Calcification Heterogeneity in Chronic Kidney Disease. Circ Res 2023;132(8):993–1012.

25. Malluche HH, Monier-Faugere MC, Blomquist G, et al. Two-year cortical and trabecular bone loss in CKD-5D: biochemical and clinical predictors. Osteoporos Int 2018;29(1):125–34.

26. Neville JJ, Palmieri T, Young AR. Physical Determinants of Vitamin D Photosynthesis: A Review. JBMR Plus 2021;5(1):e10460.

27. Baggerly CA, Cuomo RE, French CB, et al. Sunlight and Vitamin D: Necessary for Public Health. J Am Coll Nutr 2015;34(4):359–65.

28. Fantini C, Corinaldesi C, Lenzi A, et al. Vitamin D as a Shield against Aging. Int J Mol Sci 2023;24(5):4546.

29. Holick MF, Binkley NC, Bischoff-Ferrari HA, et al. Endocrine Society. Evaluation, treatment, and prevention of vitamin D deficiency: an Endocrine Society clinical practice guideline. J Clin Endocrinol Metab 2011;96(7):1911–30. Erratum in: J Clin Endocrinol Metab. 2011 Dec;96(12):3908. PMID: 21646368.

30. Orloff LA, Wiseman SM, Bernet VJ, et al. American Thyroid Association Statement on Postoperative Hypoparathyroidism: Diagnosis, Prevention, and Management in Adults. Thyroid 2018;28(7):830–41. PMID: 29848235.

31. Stack BC Jr, Bimston DN, Bodenner DL, et al. American Association Of Clinical Endocrinologists And American College Of Endocrinology Disease State Clinical Review: Postoperative Hypoparathyroidism–Definitions And Management. Endocr Pract 2015;21(6):674–85. Erratum in: Endocr Pract. 2015 Oct;21(10):1187. Dosage error in article text. PMID: 26135962.

32. Greer ML, Davis K, Stack BC Jr. Machine learning can identify patients at risk of hyperparathyroidism without known calcium and intact parathyroid hormone. Head Neck 2022;44(4):817–22. Epub 2021 Dec 25. PMID: 34953008.

33. Kato H, Hoshino Y, Hidaka N, et al. Machine Learning-Based Prediction of Elevated PTH Levels Among the US General Population. J Clin Endocrinol Metab 2022;107(12):3222–30. Erratum in: J Clin Endocrinol Metab. 2022 Dec 01;: PMID: 36125184; PMCID: PMC9693802.

34. Zhang Z, Cai L, Wu H, et al. Paricalcitol versus Calcitriol + Cinacalcet for the Treatment of Secondary Hyperparathyroidism in Chronic Kidney Disease in China: A Cost-Effectiveness Analysis. Front Public Health 2021;9:712027. PMID: 34368073; PMCID: PMC8333861.

35. Brandenburg V, Ketteler M. Vitamin D and Secondary Hyperparathyroidism in Chronic Kidney Disease: A Critical Appraisal of the Past, Present, and the Future. Nutrients 2022;14(15):3009. PMID: 35893866; PMCID: PMC9330693.

36. Parker CR, Blackwell PJ, Fairbairn KJ, et al. Alendronate in the treatment of primary hyperparathyroid-related osteoporosis: a 2-year study. J Clin Endocrinol Metab 2002;87(10):4482–9. PMID: 12364423.

37. Christodoulou M, Aspray TJ, Schoenmakers I. Vitamin D Supplementation for Patients with Chronic Kidney Disease: A Systematic Review and Meta-analyses of Trials Investigating the Response to Supplementation and an Overview of Guidelines. Calcif Tissue Int 2021;109(2):157–78. PMID: 33895867; PMCID: PMC8273061.

38. Silver Karcioglu AL, Triponez F, Solórzano CC, et al. Emerging Imaging Technologies for Parathyroid Gland Identification and Vascular Assessment in Thyroid Surgery: A

Review From the American Head and Neck Society Endocrine Surgery Section. JAMA Otolaryngol Head Neck Surg 2023;149(3):253–60. PMID: 36633855.

39. Orloff LA, Noel JE, Stack BC Jr, et al. Radiofrequency ablation and related ultrasound-guided ablation technologies for treatment of benign and malignant thyroid disease: An international multidisciplinary consensus statement of the American Head and Neck Society Endocrine Surgery Section with the Asia Pacific Society of Thyroid Surgery, Associazione Medici Endocrinologi, British Association of Endocrine and Thyroid Surgeons, European Thyroid Association, Italian Society of Endocrine Surgery Units, Korean Society of Thyroid Radiology, Latin American Thyroid Society, and Thyroid Nodules Therapies Association. Head Neck 2022;44(3):633–60. Epub 2021 Dec 23. PMID: 34939714.

Surgery for Normocalcemic Hyperparathyroidism

Pallavi Kulkarni, BS[a,b], David Goldenberg, MD, FACS[a,b,*]

KEYWORDS

- Primary hyperparathyroidism • Normocalcemic hyperparathyroidism
- Surgical management • Parathyroid

KEY POINTS

- Normocalcemic hyperparathyroidism is a phenotype of hyperparathyroidism that is becoming more prevalent due to more robust screening practices. Normocalcemic hyperparathyroidism may be an early manifestation of hypercalcemic disease. Therefore, initial diagnosis may be difficult and is one of exclusion.
- Normocalcemic hyperparathyroidism can be medically managed, and patients can be screened every 1 to 2 years if they are asymptomatic or mildly symptomatic. However, patients with clinical features and symptoms may be referred for parathyroidectomy.
- Patients with normocalcemic disease can benefit from surgery, similarly to those with hypercalcemia. However, surgical intervention can be challenging in the normocalcemic patient population due to a high rate of multiglandular involvement and small, pathologic glands. This contributes to less successful rates of complete disease eradication and increased rates of revision surgery compared to those with classical primary hyperparathyroidism.
- There is a need for longitudinal studies examining the natural history of normocalcemic primary hyperparathyroidism to better understand the value of surgery in these patients.

INTRODUCTION

Primary hyperparathyroidism (PHPT) is the most common cause of hypercalcemia, accounting for about 90% of all cases.[1] This disorder is characterized by overactive parathyroid glands, leading to increased parathyroid hormone (PTH) and excess serum calcium.[2] A different phenotype of the disease was first described in 2003, coined normocalcemic primary hyperparathyroidism (NHPT). NHPT is characterized by normal serum calcium in the face of elevated PTH. It is due to the autonomous secretion of PTH from one or more parathyroids.[3] This phenotype of PHPT has become more prevalent and recognized with increasing population screening.[4]

[a] Penn State Health Department of Otolaryngology–Head and Neck Surgery; [b] The Pennsylvania State College of Medicine, 500 University Drive, P.O. Box 850 H091 Hershey, PA 17033, USA
* Corresponding author.
E-mail address: dgoldenberg@pennstatehealth.psu.edu

Otolaryngol Clin N Am 57 (2024) 111–116
https://doi.org/10.1016/j.otc.2023.07.012
0030-6665/24/© 2023 Elsevier Inc. All rights reserved.

However, some studies suggest that NHPT may be an early form of hypercalcemic disease, with up to 20% of patients progressing to hypercalcemia.[5,6] No exact cause for NHPT development has been elucidated; however, radiation exposure is one known risk factor for NHPT.[7]

Diagnosis is challenging in these patients; NHPT is a diagnosis of exclusion. Additionally, many patients have been misclassified due to a previous lack of diagnostic criteria. Consequently, there is now a lack of knowledge of the actual prevalence and rate of complications of NHPT.[8] As outlined by the Fourth International Workshop on the Management of Asymptomatic PHPT, patients must have elevated PTH in the setting of normal albumin-corrected and ionized calcium at least 2 separate times, which should be 3 to 6 months apart.[9,10] All other causes of hyperparathyroidism should be ruled out before making an NHPT diagnosis, including but not limited to vitamin D deficiency, chronic kidney disease, medications, idiopathic hypercalciuria, and insufficient calcium intake/calcium malabsorption.[11] Most patients are found to have a biochemical profile indicative of NHPT when evaluated for clinical features or acute events such as fractures, nephrolithiasis, and osteoporosis.[12] Some clinical features maybe more severe in normocalcemic patients when compared to those with hypercalcemia. One study showed that patients with NHPT have higher rates of osteoporosis compared to those with hypercalcemia, whereas another study concluded that patients with NHPT have higher rates of nephrolithiasis compared to PHPT.[13,14]

If the patient is symptomatic, treatment in patients with NHPT can be surgical, and guidelines for asymptomatic patients can be followed for those with milder or asymptomatic disease.

Patients can be medically managed in less severe cases. Smaller pilot studies have monitored the effects of cinacalcet and bisphosphonates in NHPT, showing improvement in reducing the number and size of nephroliths and bone mineral density, respectively.[15,16] For those with more severe, symptomatic disease, surgical treatment is recommended but has added complexities involved, as there is a higher prevalence of the multiglandular disease.[17] Targeted parathyroidectomy for these patients may not be enough, and there often is a need for a 4 gland exploration and intraoperative PTH monitoring.[18]

DISCUSSION
Current Recommendations for Surgery

Parathyroidectomy for patients with hyperparathyroidism remains the mainstay for of treatment for patients with symptomatic disease or for those who are asymptomatic but meet certain criteria. However, to date, there is conflicting advice on surgical management in NHPT. The Fourth International Workshops on the Management of Asymptomatic PHPT recognized that the diagnosis was increasing but that the evidence for optimal management recommendations was insufficient.[19] Even the most recent (Fifth) Workshop on Management of PHPT has no definitive guidelines for surgery in NHPT due to limited data on long-term postoperative outcomes in this patient population.[4] It is possible that the guidelines for patients with asymptomatic PHPT may be applicable to patients with NHPT.[20] Ultimately, this leaves the decision of parathyroidectomy to the surgeon, endocrinologist and patient, evaluating whether or not the patient is likely to benefit from surgery.

Symptom and Clinical Feature Improvement

There are numerous potential benefits to surgically treating those with NHPT, especially improvements in bone mineral density. Compared to other phenotypes of hyperparathyroidism, one study showed that patients with NHPT had the most significant increase in bone mineral density at the first postoperative visit.[14] Other studies concluded that bone mineral density increased to the same degree in NHPT and hypercalcemic patients, even in those with pre-existing osteoporosis.[21,22] Aside from the clinical features often considered in patients with hyperparathyroidism, there may be some cardiovascular benefits following parathyroidectomy. In one study, NHPT and hypercalcemic patients were shown to have similarly increased cardiovascular risk factors preoperatively, such as blood pressure, lipid profiles, and glucose metabolism. However, following surgery, both groups experienced an improvement in cardiovascular risk factors, showing that PTH elevation may play a key role in disease severity.[23] The remarkable improvement seen in these patients is encouraging for the patient and surgeon.

Preoperative and Surgical Considerations

Aside from the positive endpoints after surgery, the surgeon must consider operative challenges associated with NHPT. Numerous studies have shown that NHPT is less likely to localize on imaging and is more likely to be multiglandular and manifest with smaller parathyroid glands than those seen with classic PHPT. All of this increases surgical complexity. Therefore, bilateral neck exploration may be needed for NHPT, and the need for revision surgery is more common in this patient population.[18] Monitoring of PTH after the operation can aid the surgeon in confirming successful parathyroidectomy. Still, there may be a longer time interval for a decrease in PTH levels in NHPT compared to hypercalcemic individuals.[24] All these factors can increase operative times for these patients.[8] Patients with NHPT may have an increased prevalence of recurrent and persistent disease.[14] In part, this may be due to the criteria for cure of NHPT, which involves normalization of PTH values, versus achieving eucalcemia in other phenotypes of PHPT.[25] One study showed that about 50% of the sample had persistently elevated PTH after surgery.[26] One additional consideration is that some studies show that the majority of patients with normocalcemic disease will have new concerns for nephrolithiasis following surgery, compared to classic PHPT and normohormonal PHPT patients who all had the same levels of preoperative nephrolithiasis.[14] This then questions the efficacy of parathyroidectomy for patients with NHPT, even after putting patients through a long and complex surgery compared to their hypercalcemic counterparts.

Another consideration in patients with NHPT is the utility of imaging. Preoperative localization imaging is often used in patients being considered for focused surgical treatment.[5] Current literature discusses the initial use of cervical ultrasound followed by Tc99 m radionuclide imaging. However, both ultrasound and scintigraphy are less helpful for localization in cases of NHPT. The main concern with imaging in NHPT cases is that these patients may have multiglandular disease or smaller, abnormal glands. Thus, preoperative imaging may be less sensitive.[2] In fact, in uniglandular disease, adenoma detection rates when using scintigraphy and ultrasound are comparable between normocalcemic and hypercalcemic individuals.[27] In one study, sestamibi imaging identified a single adenoma in only 14% of patients with NHPT. There are recent studies showing that 4D- CT may be superior to other forms of preoperative imaging for patients with NHPT.[28]

SUMMARY

Some patients with NHPT benefit from parathyroidectomy. However, there are important complexities in the preoperative and postoperative management of these patients, such as poor preoperative imaging localization and, thus more complex surgical planning. Surgery may have increased operative times due to multiglandular disease, a possibility for bilateral exploration, and the need for repeated intraprocedural PTH monitoring. Developing and refining appropriate imaging and preoperative planning may decrease intraoperative challenges and requirement of further extensive management. More longitudinal studies are needed to evaluate the effects of parathyroidectomy on patients with NHPT.

CLINICS CARE POINTS

- Patients with symptomatic disease should be recommended for parathyroidectomy, primarily due to the severity of clinical features seen in NHPT patients. Although there are no formal treatment guidelines, there is a need for surgical intervention, given the numerous studies that demonstrate improvement in quality of life and risk factors.

- Due to small parathyroid glands and multiglandular disease; preoperative planning remains a challenge for NHPT patients. In addition, imaging modalities that are used for hypercalcemic disease are not as sensitive for patients with NHPT. Intraoperative challenges include need for bilateral neck exploration, increased time to monitor PTH levels, and resection of multiglandular disease. This contributes to less successful rates of complete disease eradication and increased rates of revision surgery compared to those with hypercalcemic disease.

- There is a need for longitudinal studies examining the natural history of NHPT for committees and institutions to create a definitive guideline for surgical intervention.

REFERENCES

1. Minisola S, Pepe J, Piemonte S, et al. The diagnosis and management of hypercalcaemia. BMJ 2015;350(jun02 15):h2723.
2. Walker MD, Silverberg SJ. Primary hyperparathyroidism. Nat Rev Endocrinol 2018;14(2):115–25.
3. Rajkumar V, Levine SN. Normocalcemic Hyperparathyroidism. Updated 2022 Sep 3. In: StatPearls Internet. Treasure Island (FL): StatPearls Publishing; 2023-. Available from: https://www-ncbi-nlm-nih-gov.ezaccess.libraries.psu.edu/books/NBK 555967/.
4. Bilezikian JP, Khan AA, Silverberg SJ, et al. Evaluation and Management of Primary Hyperparathyroidism: Summary Statement and Guidelines from the Fifth International Workshop. J Bone Miner Res 2022;37(11):2293–314.
5. Šiprová H, Fryšák Z, Souček M. Primary hyperparathyroidism, with a focus on management of the normocalcemic form: to treat or not to treat? Endocr Pract 2016;22(3):294–301.
6. Lowe H, McMahon DJ, Rubin MR, et al. Normocalcemic primary hyperparathyroidism: further characterization of a new clinical phenotype. J Clin Endocrinol Metab 2007;92:3001–5.
7. Rao SD, Frame B, Miller MJ, et al. Hyperparathyroidism following head and neck irradiation. Arch Intern Med 1980;140(2):205–7.
8. Zavatta G, Clarke BL. Normocalcemic primary hyperparathyroidism: need for a standardized clinical approach. Endocrinology and Metabolism 2021;36: 525–35.
9. Eastell Richard, Brandi MS, Costa AG, D'Amour P, et al. Diagnosis of Asymptomatic Primary Hyperparathyroidism: Proceedings of the Fourth International

Workshop. Journal of Clinical Endocrinology & Metabolism 2014;99(Issue 10): 3570–9.

10. Schini Marian, Jacques Richard M, Oakes Eleanor, et al. Normocalcemic Hyperparathyroidism: Study of its Prevalence and Natural History. Journal of Clinical Endocrinology & Metabolism 2020;105(Issue 4):e1171–86.

11. Muñoz de Nova JL, Sampedro-Nuñez M, Huguet-Moreno I, et al. A practical approach to normocalcemic primary hyperparathyroidism. Endocrine 2021; 74(2):235–44.

12. Cusano NE, Cipriani C, Bilezikian JP. Management of normocalcemic primary hyperparathyroidism. Best Pract Res Clin Endocrinol Metab 2018;32(6):837–45.

13. Wu KCJ, Anpalahan M. Normocalcaemic primary hyperparathyroidism: is nephrolithiasis more common than osteoporosis? Intern Med J 2023;53(1):112–8.

14. Armstrong VL, Hangge PT, Butterfield R, et al. Phenotypes of primary hyperparathyroidism: Does parathyroidectomy improve clinical outcomes for all? Surgery 2023;173(1):173–9.

15. Brardi S, Cevenini G, Verdacchi T, et al. Use of cinacalcet in nephrolithiasis associated with normocalcemic or hypercalcemic primary hyperparathyroidism: results of a prospective randomized pilot study. Arch Ital Urol Androl 2015;87(1): 66–71.

16. Cesareo R, Di Stasio E, Vescini F, et al. Effects of alendronate and vitamin D in patients with normocalcemic primary hyperparathyroidism. Osteoporos Int 2015; 26(4):1295–302.

17. Choi HR, Choi SH, Hong N, et al. Comparisons Between Normocalcemic Primary Hyperparathyroidism and Typical Primary Hyperparathyroidism. J Korean Med Sci 2022;37(13):e99.

18. Pandian TK, Lubitz CC, Bird SH, et al. Normocalcemic hyperparathyroidism: a Collaborative Endocrine Surgery Quality Improvement Program analysis. Surgery 2020;167:168–72.

19. Bilezikian JP, Brandi ML, Eastell R, et al. Guidelines for the management of asymptomatic primary hyperparathyroidism: summary statement from the Fourth International Workshop. J Clin Endocrinol Metab 2014;99(10):3561–9.

20. Kulkarni P, Tucker J, King T, et al. Symptomatic versus asymptomatic primary hyperparathyroidism: A systematic review and meta-analysis. J Clin Transl Endocrinol 2023;32:100317.

21. Osorio-Silla I, Gómez-Ramírez J, Valdazo-Gómez A, et al. What happens to the bone structure after normocalcemic primary hyperparathyroidism surgery? Surgery 2022;171(4):932–9.

22. Koumakis E, Souberbielle JC, Sarfati E, et al. Bone mineral density evolution after successful parathyroidectomy in patients with normocalcemic primary hyperparathyroidism. J Clin Endocrinol Metab 2013;98(8):3213–20.

23. Beysel S, Caliskan M, Kizilgul M, et al. Parathyroidectomy improves cardiovascular risk factors in normocalcemic and hypercalcemic primary hyperparathyroidism. BMC Cardiovasc Disord 2019;19(1):106.

24. Graves CE, McManus CM, Chabot JA, et al. Biochemical profile affects IOPTH kinetics and cure rate in primary hyperparathyroidism. World J Surg 2020;44: 488–95.

25. Wilhelm SM, Wang TS, Ruan DT, et al. The American Association of Endocrine Surgeons Guidelines for Definitive Management of Primary Hyperparathyroidism. JAMA Surg 2016;151(10):959–68.

26. Sho S, Kuo EJ, Chen AC, et al. Biochemical and Skeletal Outcomes of Parathy-roidectomy for Normocalcemic (Incipient) Primary Hyperparathyroidism. Ann Surg Oncol 2019;26:539–46.
27. Wade TJ, Yen TWF, Amin AL, et al. Surgical management of normocalcemic pri-mary hyperparathyroidism. World J Surg 2012;6:761–6.
28. Cunha-Bezerra P, Vieira R, Amaral F, et al. Better performance of four-dimension computed tomography as a localization procedure in normocalcemic primary hy-perparathyroidism. J Med Imaging Radiat Oncol 2018;62(4):493–8.

Parathyroidectomy
An Operative Guide

Catherine Alessandra Colaianni, MD, MPhil[a], Maisie Shindo, MD[b],*

KEYWORDS

- Parathyroidectomy • Parathyroid hormone • Subtotal parathyroidectomy
- Four-gland exploration

KEY POINTS

- With proper preparation, parathyroidectomy can be a straightforward and safe operation.
- Intraoperative decision-making regarding multiglandular disease should be based on visual inspection of all 4 glands and intraoperative parathyroid hormone levels. Intraoperative pathology consultation or autofluorescence technology can also be useful if available.
- Taking care to preserve the inferior thyroid artery can prevent inadvertent devascularization of the inferior parathyroid glands.

INTRODUCTION

Parathyroidectomy can be aptly summarized with the first sentence of Charles Dickens' canonical novel, *A Tale of Two Cities*: it can be the best of times, and the worst of times. A relatively straightforward and satisfying operation can become a dreaded one with improper preparation, decision-making, or technique. Herein, we describe our approach to targeted parathyroidectomy and 4 gland exploration for primary hyperparathyroidism. Elsewhere in this issue are sections devoted to the management of 4 gland hyperplasia, secondary hyperparathyroidism, normocalcemic hyperparathyroidism, and ectopic or difficult-to-locate glands; therefore, though the content herein is relevant to the management of those clinical issues, they are not the primary focus of this study.

PREOPERATIVE PATIENT EDUCATION AND INFORMED CONSENT

In informed consent discussions with patients undergoing parathyroidectomy, discussion of risks should include damage to the recurrent laryngeal nerve that can result in

[a] Otolaryngology–Head and Neck Surgery, Oregon Health and Science University;
[b] Department of Otolaryngology, Head and Neck Surgery, Head & Neck Endocrine Surgery, Oregon Health and Science University, 3181 Southwest Sam Jackson Park Road, Portland OR 97239, USA
* Corresponding author. 3181 Southwest Sam Jackson Park Road, Portland, OR 97214.
E-mail address: shindom@ohsu.edu

Otolaryngol Clin N Am 57 (2024) 117–123
https://doi.org/10.1016/j.otc.2023.08.004
0030-6665/24/© 2023 Elsevier Inc. All rights reserved.

changes to voice and swallowing, need for temporary or permanent supplemental calcium and/or vitamin D postoperatively, and need for reoperation. Depending on our preoperative suspicion of intrathyroidal parathyroid adenoma, or of parathyroid carcinoma, consent for possible concomitant hemi or total thyroidectomy and/or central/paratracheal neck dissection may need to be added.

PREOPERATIVE DISCUSSION WITH ANESTHESIOLOGY TEAM
Monitored Anesthesia Care Versus General Anesthetic

In certain cases, such as a well-localized single adenoma, or a single adenoma in an individual who requires parathyroidectomy but is unable to undergo general anesthesia due to medical comorbidities, monitored anesthesia care with local anesthetic may be appropriate in lieu of general endotracheal anesthesia.[1] In appropriate cases, this has the added benefit of decreasing nonoperative times during parathyroid surgery.[2]

Endotracheal Tube/Intubation

Although the use of intraoperative nerve monitoring for thyroidectomy is widely accepted, its use is somewhat controversial for routine parathyroidectomy. Indications for its use in parathyroidectomy are prior surgery in or near the operative field and parathyroid tumors in a location that may require significant dissection of the recurrent laryngeal nerve, such as an inferiorly and posteriorly located superior gland where the nerve may course anterior to the adenoma. Should nerve monitoring be used, the surgeon should confirm correct tube placement.

Intravenous Placement

Anticipating multiple intraoperative blood draws to assess parathyroid hormone (PTH) levels, it is recommended that a second, large-bore intravenous (IV) specifically for repeat blood draws be placed.

Patient Positioning

1. Patients undergoing parathyroidectomy should be positioned supine, with one or both arms tucked in a way that permits the anesthesiologist to access upper extremity IV lines for intraoperative blood draws.
2. Turning the operating table 90 or 180° for 4 gland exploration can be helpful for retractor placement particularly to access the lower neck and mediastinum. In cases with a well-localized target gland, keeping the head of the bed toward anesthesia can also be appropriate.
3. In patients with adequate neck mobility and without cervical disc disease, a small shoulder or axillary gel pad can be placed to aid in neck extension. In addition, a rolled towel under the neck can be placed for added support to minimize postoperative posterior neck pain.

Intraoperative Ultrasound

Intraoperative ultrasound is a useful adjunct for targeted parathyroidectomy.[3] After positioning, we favor utilizing intraoperative ultrasound for incision planning, target gland confirmation, and planning anterior versus lateral approach. Particularly for patients with neck mobility issues or anterior neck pain preventing using adequate pressure on the transducer to permit visualization of deeper or paraesophageal adenomas, using the ultrasound effectively in the clinic may be challenging. Repeating the ultrasound under general anesthesia allows greater pressure to be applied with the transducer to improve examination of more posteriorly located areas to relocalize (or localize) candidate adenomas. If a candidate adenoma is identified, its location is marked to determine the incision placement.

Incision Placement

If a candidate adenoma is identified, a low collar incision over the location of the adenoma in an existing skin crease is preferred (**Fig. 1**). Length of the incision varies depending on the location and size of the adenoma as well as the preoperative likelihood of bilateral exploration. Incision length may range from 3 to approximately 5 cm, with extension for patients with limited neck mobility, prior anterior neck surgery, or deep adenomas. After marking the incision, local anesthetic is injected to minimize the need for intraoperative narcotic pain medication given by the anesthesia team.

Preoperative Labs

Before the start of the operation, a baseline intraoperative PTH level should be drawn.

OPERATIVE STEPS FOR TARGETED PARATHYROIDECTOMY

1. The incision is made sharply with a scalpel through the skin and subcutaneous fat.
2. The platysma is divided sharply or with electrocautery.
3. Subplatysmal flaps are raised superiorly and inferiorly.
4. A self-retaining retractor is placed vertically into the wound (**Fig. 2**).
5. Four hook retractors are placed in the 4 quadrants of the wound to retract the skin.
6. Anterior approach:
   a. The midline raphe is identified and divided using electrocautery.
   b. The sternohyoid and sternothyroid muscles on the side of the target gland are reflected laterally off of the thyroid gland. Often this step can be performed bluntly using a Freer elevator (**Fig. 3**).
   c. For inferior glands, the inferior thyroid lobe is retracted medially using a Babcock or Kittner sponge, and the fibrofatty tissue near the gland is gently dissected until the candidate adenoma is identified (**Fig. 4**).
   d. For superior glands, the superolateral aspect of the thyroid gland is retracted medially using a Babcock or Kittner sponge. Fibrofatty tissue adjacent to the thyroid gland is gently dissected until the candidate adenoma is identified.

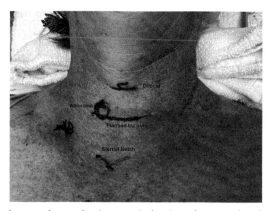

Fig. 1. Suspected adenoma located using postinduction ultrasound. Adenoma location (*circle*), cricoid, sternal notch, and planned incision.

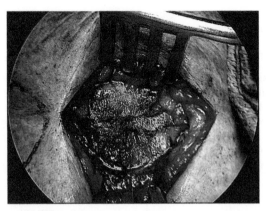

Fig. 2. Weitlaner retractor placed.

7. Alternative: lateral approach. Our senior author has described a lateral approach, which minimizes dissection of the thyroid gland and which we prefer for deep, retroesophageal, paraesophageal, or superior adenomas that may be accessed between the sternocleidomastoid muscle and strap muscles.[4] This approach is not routine in most practices, and deep, retroesophageal, paraesophageal, or superior adenomas may be safely accessed using the anterior approach described above.
   a. The anterior border of the sternocleidomastoid muscle is identified low, unwrapped and retracted laterally, exposing the lateral border of the strap muscles.
   b. The strap muscles, together with the ansa hypoglossi nerve are retracted medially and the internal jugular vein and carotid artery are identified and gently retracted laterally.
   c. The thyroid capsule is exposed deep to the strap muscles and is retracted medially together with the strap muscles, allowing visualization and access to the posterolateral thyroid and tracheoesophageal groove.
8. Once the candidate adenoma is identified, it can usually be bluntly dissected free from surrounding tissue using a Freer elevator, using bipolar electrocautery on the polar vessels and on small vessels along the capsule (**Fig. 5**). Note: If the adenoma is not able to be easily dissected using a Freer elevator, or is adherent to the

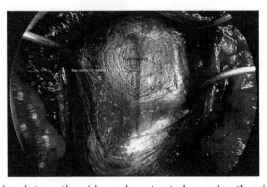

Fig. 3. Sternohyoid and sternothyroid muscles retracted exposing thyroid capsule.

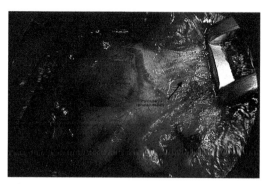

Fig. 4. Thyroid tubercle grasped with Babcock clamp, retracted medially exposing inferior parathyroid adenoma.

surrounding tissue, the recurrent laryngeal nerve should be identified before division or cauterization of surrounding tissue to reduce the risk of inadvertent injury. Note: Care must be taken not to compress, crush, or traumatize the gland as this can lead to falsely elevated parathyroid hormone levels, and worse, rupture of the gland which can result in seeding of parathyroid cells and recurrence (parathyromatosis).

9. Once the gland is removed, if it does not look like a classic adenoma, or if our clinical suspicion is high for parathyroid carcinoma, we send the gland for frozen pathology to confirm hypercellular parathyroid tissue.
10. Once the gland is removed, intraoperative PTH levels should be drawn at 10 and 15 minutes postremoval.
11. If the PTH level drops appropriately (< 50% of baseline, and within the normal range), the wound is checked for hemostasis and closed.
12. If the PTH level does not drop appropriately, the remaining gland on the ipsilateral side should be identified. If the second identified gland appears normal, it can be confirmed by performing frozen section of a small fragment with tenotomy scissors to confirm parathyroid tissue. If biopsy is performed, it should be carefully taken from the part of the gland that is furthest away from its blood supply. Whether or not it is hypercellular or normal can be difficult for the pathologist to differentiate. An alternative to biopsy for confirmation of parathyroid gland is

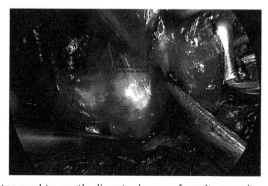

Fig. 5. Freer elevator used to gently dissect adenoma from its capsule.

autofluorescence technology.[5] If the pathologist is unable to determine relative cellularity, the decision to excise the gland will need to be based on its size rather than its cellularity. A gland may be mildly hypercellular but normal in size due to concurrent secondary hyperparathyroidism such as chronic vitamin D deficiency. Similarly, a parathyroid gland may be mildly enlarged, but not be hyperfunctional.[6] Therefore, it should only be removed if it is enlarged and not before identifying additional glands. If multiglandular pathology is entertained, the patient's contralateral side should be explored and inspected in the same manner as detailed above before any additional glands are excised. The rationale for this is that the decision should be made as to which gland will be best left in-situ in the patient to minimize risk of permanent hypoparathyroidism (see section on bilateral exploration).

13. The wound may then be closed in layers. For bilateral explorations, a suction drain may be used to prevent seroma.
14. We favor the use of additional local anesthetic agents at the conclusion of the case to minimize the need for postoperative narcotics for pain management.

OPERATIVE PEARLS FOR BILATERAL OR FOUR-GLAND EXPLORATION

1. If there is no candidate gland on preoperative ultrasound and other localization studies, particularly in complex or revision cases, one way we determine which side to start on is to take preoperative PTH samples from both internal jugular veins.
2. The first important principle in bilateral exploration is understanding the typical and ectopic locations of parathyroid glands.
3. The second important principle is preservation of the blood supply to each parathyroid gland. It is imperative that the blood supply to the parathyroid glands be protected so as not to inadvertently devascularize the parathyroid glands. The surgeon should be cognizant of the variation in blood supply (polar vessel) to parathyroid glands. For example, the polar vessel to the inferior gland is not always on the lateral surface of the parathyroid gland but sometimes can course to the thyroid capsule above the parathyroid gland and then course back laterally to the medial aspect of the parathyroid gland. Thus small vessels lateral to the thyroid or surrounding the parathyroid should not be ligated or cauterized as these could be feeding the parathyroid glands (**Fig. 6**).

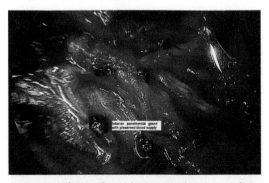

Fig. 6. Relationship between inferior thyroid artery and recurrent laryngeal nerve. Inferior parathyroid gland with preserved blood supply. Ligating the artery lateral to the branch to the inferior gland will preserve the gland.

4. The third important principle is to inspect all 4 glands before excision if hyperplasia is suspected. After identification, if only 2 glands are enlarged (double adenoma), the two abnormal glands should be excised and PTH levels drawn after excision. If 3 glands are abnormal, all 3 should be excised, leaving a well-vascularized fourth. With 4 gland hyperplasia, at least 3 glands are excised, and an appropriate portion of the 4th gland is left in situ. If we are considering autotransplantation for any reason, we send a fragment of the gland to be autotransplanted for frozen section to confirm parathyroid tissue. With 4 gland hyperplasia, the decision regarding which gland should be left behind is based on the viability of the gland, and the most vascularized gland should be selected to be left behind, in part or in total. For this reason, it cannot be over-emphasized that the blood supply to each gland be protected during the initial exploration, as the determination of which gland will be left behind will be made after inspecting all 4. Injury to the blood supply of the gland that will ultimately need to be left behind can result in permanent hypoparathyroidism. If 2 glands appear equally vascularized, the decision for which gland to leave in situ can also factor in location of the gland. In this situation, we prefer to leave the gland not in close proximity to the recurrent laryngeal nerve, should the patient need reoperative surgery in the future.

DISCLOSURE

Dr C.A. Colaianni and Dr M. Shindo have no financial disclosures or conflicts of interest to report.

REFERENCES

1. Starker LF, Fonseca AL, Carling T, et al. Minimally invasive parathyroidectomy. Int J Endocrinol 2011;206502.
2. Iwata AJ, Wertz Anna S, Alluri Spandana, et al. A faster parathyroidectomy: Techniques to shorten non-surgical operating room time. Am J Otolaryngol 2019;40(6).
3. Butt HZ, Husainy MA, Bolia A, et al. Ultrasonography alone can reliably locate parathyroid tumours and facilitates minimally invasive parathyroidectomy. Ann R Coll Surg Engl 2015;97(6):420–4.
4. Shindo ML, Rosenthal JM. Minimal Access Parathyroidectomy Using the Focused Lateral Approach: Technique, Indication, and Results. Arch Otolaryngol Head Neck Surg 2007;133(12):1227–34.
5. Silver Karcioglu AL, Triponez F, Solórzano CC, et al. Emerging Imaging Technologies for Parathyroid Gland Identification and Vascular Assessment in Thyroid Surgery: A Review From the American Head and Neck Society Endocrine Surgery Section. JAMA Otolaryngol Head Neck Surg 2023;149(3):253–60.
6. Sekine O, Hozumi Y, Takemoto N, et al. Parathyroid adenoma without hyperparathyroidism. Jpn J Clin Oncol 2004;34(3):155–8.

Pearls of Parathyroidectomy
How to Find the Hard to Find Ones

Zoe H. Fullerton, MD, MBE, Lisa A. Orloff, MD*

KEYWORDS

- Primary hyperparathyroidism • Nonlocalized • Parathyroidectomy
- Multigland disease • Elusive

KEY POINTS

- Preparation is essential: know or suspect as much as possible *before* you go to the operating room (OR).
- Imaging is highly variable and operator-dependent—do it/review it yourself.
- Keep a dry surgical field from the outset and dissect sequentially, not skipping areas.
- Lesions are commonly *deeper* than expected—dissect to the prevertebral plane if necessary.
- If intraoperative parathyroid hormone does not drop, do not remove serially identified parathyroid glands after the first until all other glands are identified and compared.

 Video content accompanies this article at http://www.oto.theclinics.com.

INTRODUCTION

Few situations are more frustrating to a parathyroid surgeon than undertaking surgery for primary hyperparathyroidism (PHPT) where, despite best attempts preoperatively and intraoperatively, the offending gland(s) are not located and the patient's disease remains. Sooner or later, even the most experienced parathyroid surgeon will experience this scenario, which underscores the importance of using a comprehensive and systematic approach to identifying parathyroid lesions. By doing so, surgeons can maximize cure while minimizing exasperation and complications.

CLINICAL EVALUATION

The first step in evaluating a patient with PHPT is confirming the diagnosis. PHPT is characterized by elevated parathyroid hormone (PTH) levels with concurrent

Department of Otolaryngology–Head and Neck Surgery, Stanford University, 801 Welch Road, Stanford, CA 94305, USA
* Corresponding author.
E-mail address: lorloff@stanford.edu

Otolaryngol Clin N Am 57 (2024) 125–137
https://doi.org/10.1016/j.otc.2023.07.004
0030-6665/24/© 2023 Elsevier Inc. All rights reserved.

oto.theclinics.com

hypercalcemia or inappropriate normocalcemia. Other potential etiologies such as vitamin D toxicity, vitamin D deficiency, medication use, familial hypercalcemic hypocalciuria, or renal disease should have been considered and addressed before recommending surgery. It is also crucial to consider comorbidities that increase the likelihood of multiglandular disease (MGD), such as multiple endocrine neoplasia type 1, lithium use, and chronic renal disease.

Once the diagnosis is confirmed, one should assess the condition's severity and understand the patient's expectations and goals. If the patient is symptomatic (eg, history of renal calculi, complications of osteoporosis), timely surgical intervention should be discussed. For asymptomatic patients and those identified early in their course of disease, observation may be considered, particularly when a candidate lesion is not apparent. Anatomical challenges such as concurrent thyroid disease or prior anterior neck surgery should be noted. Similarly, significant cervical adiposity, kyphosis or other limits in neck extension and other comorbidities should be considered. Knowing whether a patient has a history of Hashimoto's thyroiditis, goiter, or thyroid nodularity is necessary for operative planning and for guiding further assessment and care. For patients referred for revision surgery, one should review prior surgical reports and consider additional studies to maximize understanding of anatomy and identify potential residual sources of disease.

PREOPERATIVE IMAGING

The increased preference for minimally invasive parathyroidectomy over bilateral neck exploration has made preoperative imaging and localization essential to surgical planning. It is imperative to review all available images personally and conduct any confirmatory studies before proceeding with surgical intervention. Each imaging modality varies in the data that it provides. To appropriately use these tools, a surgeon must understand each study's limitations and exercise clinical judgment when interpreting findings.

Parathyroid Ultrasound

Ultrasound is the most cost-effective and often the first-line imaging modality for parathyroid disease. The skill and experience of the sonographer often determine the results of these studies, which can lead to variable sensitivity in parathyroid adenoma (PTA) detection, with rates ranging from 53% to 93%.[1,2] Most high-volume thyroid and parathyroid centers tend to achieve higher rates.

Ultrasound provides information on pathology as well as surgical anatomy. A surgeon trained in ultrasonography can confirm or challenge previous imaging studies. Clinical ultrasound can be used to identify a suspected PTA, its relationship to nearby structures, and coexistent thyroid pathology. Office-based ultrasound is reliable in localizing PTAs in 90% of cases and is more sensitive in detecting sub-centimeter adenomas when compared with radionuclide imaging.[3]

Techniques for Ultrasound Identification

A systematic and complete ultrasound examination should be performed for every patient, regardless of whether separate imaging has suggested one or more candidate lesions. A comprehensive ultrasound survey provides a complete understanding of the target lesion, its surrounding anatomy, and the presence of any concurrent lesions, anatomic abnormalities, or MGD. PTAs are generally best detected with a high-frequency transducer (7.5–12 MHz). They usually appear as well-circumscribed, oval, hypoechoic lesions distinct from the thyroid capsule (**Fig. 1**, Videos 1 and 2).

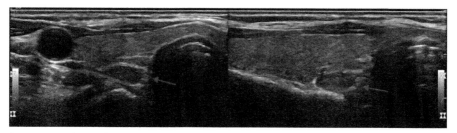

Fig. 1. Typical parathyroid adenoma (*red arrows*; ultrasound, right transverse [*left panel*], and sagittal [*right panel*] views).

Occasionally, they have a bilobed or lobulated shape. PTAs are highly vascular lesions with a "feeding artery" entering at the long axis, typically branching from the inferior thyroid artery. Power Doppler may reveal intense peripheral and polar flow (**Fig. 2**, Video 3).

The entire neck should be examined, including lateral neck compartments. Scan of the central neck should include adjustments performed by the patient (head-turning, swallowing, hyperextension) and the examiner (adjusting ultrasound frequency, gain, and depth, applying variable pressure to the transducer, incorporating Doppler, and so forth).[4] The examination should begin with close inspection of the most common anatomic locations of the parathyroid glands. The areas posterior and inferior to the inferior edge of the thyroid should be inspected for inferior glands, and the region posterior to the mid-portion extending to the superior pole should be inspected for superior glands. The entire depth of the field from the strap muscles to the prevertebral fascia should be inspected; examination should be continued as inferiorly as possible into the thymic and superior mediastinal regions. Parathyroid lesions tend to enlarge in an inferior direction from their host gland, and the so-called "descended" parathyroids can be located quite deep and inferior in the neck (**Fig. 3**). Understanding the relationship of the lesion to the thyroid gland, middle thyroid vein, inferior thyroid artery, esophagus, cricoid, clavicle, and strap muscles is essential, as these can provide landmarks during surgery. Although vascular anomalies are rare, they may suggest anatomic aberrations in parathyroid locations.[5] The absence of a normal innominate artery bifurcation into subclavian and carotid arteries implies a nonrecurrent right inferior laryngeal nerve and the potential for ectopic parathyroid gland positioning.

If no candidate lesion is identified, inspecting the piriform sinus, retroesophageal, and retrotracheal areas is attempted. However, these areas and those behind bony structures are less accessible to ultrasound examination, and lesions here may elude detection.

Regardless of central compartment findings, an examination of the lateral neck on both sides should then be conducted. Supernumerary or anatomically aberrant glands may be identified, especially within the carotid sheath. Distinguishing parathyroid lesions from lymph nodes can be challenging, but Doppler identification of a hilar pattern versus a polar inflow or diffuse flow can help. In these cases, fine needle aspiration (FNA) with PTH washout in addition to cytology may be indicated, especially if malignant lymphadenopathy is in the differential diagnosis (see below).

Nuances of Parathyroid Ultrasound

Because of variability in the migration patterns of parathyroids during embryonic development, superior and inferior glands do not always end up in their expected

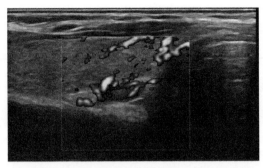

Fig. 2. Parathyroid adenoma, ultrasound with power Doppler demonstrating polar feeding artery and diffuse vascularity (right sagittal view).

positions. However, the relative depth of the glands and relationship to the recurrent laryngeal nerve (RLN) tends to be constant. Superior parathyroids are typically located deep or dorsal to the RLN; inferior glands are superficial or ventral to the RLN. Observing the angle of the structure in the sagittal plane can provide clues to the origin of the gland. Superior parathyroids often point deep, with the inferior edge extending dorsally parallel to the vertebrae. Conversely, inferior glands often point superficial toward the strap muscles (**Fig. 4**). Although it is generally thought that normal parathyroid glands are not identifiable on ultrasound, careful attention to subtle variations in echogenicity can sometimes reveal normal parathyroid glands as small, homogenously hyperechoic, nodular structures (**Fig. 5**). The identification of a normal gland strongly decreases the likelihood of MGD.[6]

Even if a candidate lesion has been found, the ultrasound examination should continue to assess for potential MGD (including double adenoma) and to avoid being misled by imposter structures (**Fig. 6**). Yet if a candidate lesion is not identified despite all the above maneuvers, one should consider other localization techniques, such as those discussed below.

Sestamibi Radionuclide Imaging

Gamma-ray imaging is a functional modality for hyperparathyroidism that can be used with or without concurrent single-photon emission computed tomography (SPECT). The most common agent, Technetium Tc99 m sestamibi, is administered through

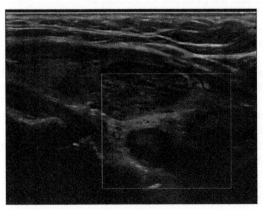

Fig. 3. Descended right superior parathyroid adenoma (sagittal ultrasound with power Doppler) in the prevertebral plane.

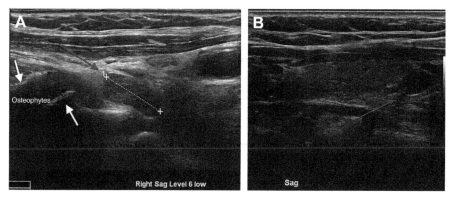

Fig. 4. (*A*) Superior parathyroid adenomas tend to point deep at their inferior aspect on sagittal view (*red arrow*); (*B*) inferior adenomas tend to point superficially at their inferior aspect on sagittal view (*red arrow*).

intravenous injection. Sequential images are then obtained to visualize uptake and washout of the isotope. Planar images are taken at 10- and 90- to 120-minute intervals. PTAs tend to have delayed washout and may be identifiable in later images (**Fig. 7**).

The addition of SPECT directly after the planar images allows the lesions to be localized in three dimensions. The combination of SPECT and CT requires additional radiation exposure but provides better anatomic characterization of the lesions (**Fig. 8**). Meta-analysis has found that the sensitivity of sestamibi is 63% and SPECT is 79%.[7,8] The integration of these two modalities with CT increases the sensitivity to 84%.[8,9] Smaller size PTAs, those with high washout rates (15%–40% of all adenomas), and MGD is often undetected.[7] This results in a high false-negative rate (as much as 20%) for the procedure.[2,8] Nevertheless, a negative sestamibi scan is informative, as it raises the suspicion for small or multigland disease, and tends to rule out a mediastinal lesion that would have been missed on ultrasound. Like ultrasound, sestamibi scanning is also operator- and interpreter-dependent. If images are obtained at

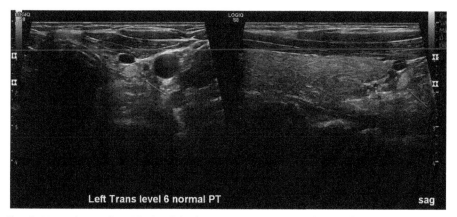

Fig. 5. Normal parathyroid gland (*red arrows*, transverse [*left panel*] and sagittal [*right panel*] B-mode ultrasound).

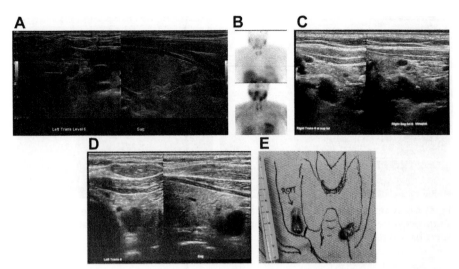

Fig. 6. All of the following were from a patient with a single parathyroid adenoma. (*A*) Imposter (*red arrows*) that proved to be a benign lymph node (despite lack of visible hilum on ultrasound). (*B*) Planar sestamibi scan suggesting right inferior parathyroid adenoma. (*C*) Intraoperative (before incision) ultrasound suggesting right superior parathyroid lesion (note pointing deep on sagittal view). (*D*) Intraoperative ultrasound, reidentifying left-sided imposter. (*E*) Surgical specimens. The right-sided lesion was deep/dorsal to the RLN, IOPTH of aspirate was >5000 pg/mL, and final pathology confirmed parathyroid adenoma. The left-sided lesion was ventral to the RLN, IOPTH of aspirate was 7 pg/mL (> serum level, ie, non-parathyroid source), and final pathology-confirmed benign lymph node.

too long of an interval, washout may have already occurred, and a false negative result may occur. A detail-oriented nuclear medicine service will perform washout scanning sequentially between and after the 10- and 120-minute views. The surgeon should review all sestamibi images regardless of the official reading, as subtle lesions may be identifiable that are not reported.

The histological makeup of a parathyroid lesion may affect its ability to be detected on a sestamibi scan. Adenomas are predominated by either chief cells or oxyphil cells. Studies have shown that oxyphil cells, which have higher concentrations of mitochondria, take up more sestamibi. Therefore, adenomas with a lower ratio of oxyphil cells have lower rates of uptake and quicker washout, which may result in a false negative scan.[9]

Four-Dimensional Computed Tomography /Four-Dimensional MRI

Four-dimensional computed tomography (4D-CT) is a technique that exploits the differential rate of contrast washout between PTAs and surrounding tissues. The 3D CT scan is augmented by capturing images at various stages of contrast washout over the fourth dimension time (**Fig. 9**). Although the 4D-CT has been shown to have a sensitivity of up to 87% for PTAs, it requires the specialized expertise of trained neuroradiologists and technicians for accurate results.[1,2,10] Thyroid nodules, background thyroiditis, cystic change, and hemorrhage may make detection less reliable.[11,12] Importantly, the radiation dose delivered to the thyroid by 4D-CT is more than 50 times higher than that delivered with sestamibi which should be considered in its use, especially with younger individuals.[13]

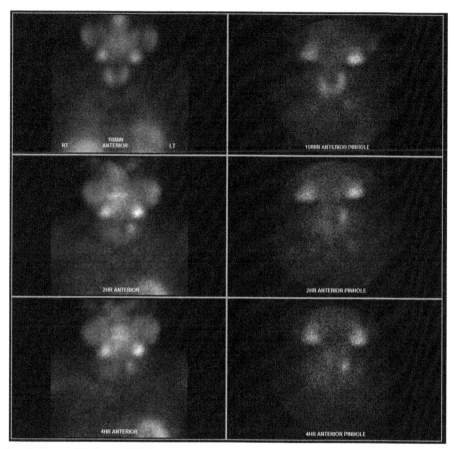

Fig. 7. Sestamibi planar (2D) images; early (10 minutes), late (2 hours), and later (4 hours), showing thyroid washout with time and retention in a left superior parathyroid adenoma.

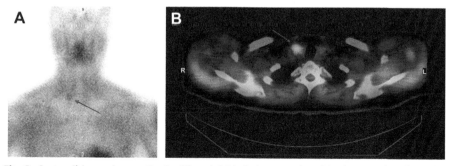

Fig. 8. Sestamibi scan in a patient with a right inferior parathyroid adenoma (confirmed at surgery). (*A*) Planar tomograms showing subtle retention in the right inferior region (*red arrow*). (*B*) SPECT/CT, axial view, showing more obvious retention in a right inferior lesion (*red arrow*).

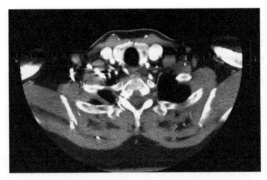

Fig. 9. 4D-CT, axial view, showing a right superior parathyroid candidate lesion (*red arrow*) with contrast enhancement on early (arterial phase) imaging.

A similar protocol has been developed with MRI. 4D-MRI uses the unique magnetic resonance perfusion characteristics of PTAs to identify lesions. It particularly has been shown to have a high degree of accuracy (85%) in identification of double adenomas.[14] Although this technique mitigates the radiation concerns of 4D-CT, the limited availability of the 3 T MR scanners and required expertise in the unique protocols limit its accessibility.[15]

18F-Fluorocholine PET/Computed Tomography and PET/MRI

A recent addition to parathyroid imaging is PET/CT or PET/MRI with the radiopharmaceutical 18F-fluorocholine (FCH). Uptake of FCH is higher in cells with hyperproliferation or increased intracellular metabolism such as PTAs (**Fig. 10**). Although access to this technique is still limited, it has been shown to have 81% sensitivity for previously nonlocalized adenomas. This technique has also shown promising sensitivity in small-volume studies for patients with familial and multiple gland disease.[16,17]

OTHER LOCALIZATION STUDIES
Parathyroid Fine Needle Aspiration

Ultrasound-guided preoperative (or intraoperative) parathyroid FNA is a technique that can be used to confirm the parathyroid origin of detected candidate lesions in challenging anatomic fields (previously operated, intrathyroidal, non-concordant imaging studies, and so forth). The smallest gauge needle should be used and the needle washout with saline should be sent for PTH chemistry testing which is more reliable

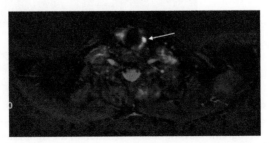

Fig. 10. FCH PET MRI, axial view, demonstrating left inferior parathyroid adenoma (*white arrow*) that was paraesophageal.

than parathyroid cytology. Unequivocally, high levels of PTH are detected if the source is a parathyroid gland (> background circulating serum levels, usually by at least an order of magnitude). This technique should be used sparingly as there is a theoretical possibility of implanting parathyroid cells in surrounding tissue and potential for fibrosis and inflammatory response, which can increase surgical complexity.[18]

Venous Sampling

Selective venous sampling for PTH concentrations is another technique to consider in cases where a candidate cannot be identified. This process compares venous concentrations of PTH from different sites to establish laterality for the likely adenoma. It can be performed with ultrasound-guided bilateral internal jugular vein sampling or interventional radiology performed multisite "super-selective" sampling. Meta-analysis shows that "super-selective" sampling has higher sensitivity and accuracy, with sensitivities ranging from 75% to 93%.[19] Although the invasiveness of this technique does not lend itself to routine cases, it may be considered in situations where multiple other modalities have been unsuccessful.

What If I Still Cannot Find It?

If there is no disease localization despite multiple studies, the surgeon should hypothesize that the patient has MGD and plan accordingly. Careful notation of the bilateral neck anatomy on ultrasound is beneficial when anticipating a bilateral neck exploration. It is also essential to counsel the patient about an increased risk of complications and disease persistence, especially in a revision or reattempt at excision.

INTRAOPERATIVE APPROACHES TO PARATHYROID IDENTIFICATION

As with many surgical procedures, those who perform a larger number of parathyroidectomies are more likely to have lower rates of complications and higher success rates.[20] Parathyroid surgery has an overall estimated success rate of 95% to 99%.[21] However, for even the most experienced surgeon, a non-localized parathyroid case presents a challenge. Subtle variants of HPT, such as normohormonal and normocalcemic HPT, present added challenges. In these and all parathyroid cases, certain measures should be taken to ensure the maximal chance of success while minimizing risk.

Preparation

A careful review of previous operative and pathology reports cannot be overemphasized. Repeating ultrasonography in the operating room before incision allows the clinician to be prepared to navigate a patient's specific anatomy. Inserting an esophageal probe can be helpful for deep or paraesophageal lesions as the probe often displaces PTAs superficially. This can be tested under ultrasound with the option of removal if the lesion's new position is not more easily accessible (**Fig. 11**, Video 4). An accurate measurement of preoperative PTH levels and obtaining intraoperative PTH (IOPTH) can help determine operative success; this process often requires close collaboration with the anesthesia team.

Intraoperative

Incision placement is critical to ensure access to relevant anatomy. An incision placed too high will limit access to the thymus and upper mediastinum. An incision positioned too low will limit access to the superior glands. Although an off-center incision may be ideal for lateral access to a well-localized superior PTA, when there is any doubt about

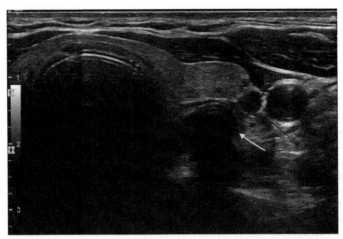

Fig. 11. Transverse ultrasound in the operating room before incision, showing esophageal temperature probe (*yellow arrow*) displacing a left inferior parathyroid adenoma to a more lateral and superficial location (*red arrow*).

the number or location of affected glands, a low transverse midline incision generally allows for the best surgical access. Although concern for cosmetic outcomes often motivates using small incisions, one should not hesitate to enlarge an incision for adequate surgical visualization.

Additional surgical aids include loupe magnification, the use of a headlight, and adjustable retraction. An assistant applying excessive retraction may be counterproductive and runs the risk of exerting traction forces that can translate to the RLN. Intraoperative nerve monitoring, when available, can decrease likelihood of bilateral vocal fold paralysis by allowing the clinician to confirm preserved nerve signals on one dissection side before proceeding to the other.

Parathyroid surgery aims to expose and retrieve the offending gland(s) while limiting trauma to surrounding tissues including normal parathyroid glands. It is vital to maintain stringent hemostasis, as color contrast is essential in parathyroid identification. The procedure should begin on the side of the most likely offending gland. If a four-gland exploration is needed, one should first expose and identify each gland. This limits the possibility of unintentionally excising all normal parathyroid glands and being left with only the final abnormal gland.

If an inferior or ventral lesion is suspected, it may not be necessary to expose the ipsilateral RLN, which will run deep to the lesion. If a superior parathyroid lesion is suspected, the surgeon should anticipate dissecting dorsal to the RLN, increasing the likelihood that the nerve will require identification and dissection. For very deep superior lesions, dissection medial to the carotid artery down to the prevertebral plane may allow delivery of the lesion without encountering the RLN; in this setting, nerve monitoring and testing the vagus nerve for stimulation can confirm preservation of RLN integrity even without its exposure.

To maximize the preservation of normal thyroid and parathyroid glands, the superior and inferior thyroid arteries should be preserved whenever possible; smaller vessels can be divided and ligated to medially rotate the thyroid gland and allow access to deep and medial neck spaces. Tracing the inferior thyroid artery to its terminal branches that enter the thyroid gland can help lead to the parathyroid glands. The tubercle of Zuckerkandl is a useful thyroid landmark that assists in localizing the RLN; however, the tubercle can also be easily mistaken for a parathyroid lesion. Other imposters include lobulations of thyroid tissue, central compartment lymph nodes (common in Hashimoto's thyroiditis), and brown fat.

Dissection should be conducted in a continuous linear fashion within any given region. Skipping between levels increases the risk of missing a lesion in intervening layers. Extracapsular thyroid dissection provides access to deeper layers. Often, a suspected lesion proves to be deeper in vivo, especially after displacement of retracted anatomy, than it appeared on pre-incision imaging. If the immediate tissue in contact with the thyroid has been explored, dissection should outline the boundaries of level 6, using the carotid and innominate arteries and spine to identify and preserve the RLNs and esophagus while revealing adjacent parathyroid glands.

Measuring IOPTH after excision of a target can help determine whether the tissue was the source of disease. Needle aspiration and PTH washout of the excised tissue can help differentiate a parathyroid candidate from non-parathyroid structures. Parathyroid autofluorescence can also help identify parathyroid glands. Normal and hyperplastic parathyroid tissue usually fluoresces at least 1.5 to 2.0 times more and often much greater than the background thyroid. In contrast, the difference between a PTA and thyroid tissue is less, likely due to defective calcium-sensing machinery in the neoplastic tissue.

If the above techniques have been applied, ipsilateral RLN integrity and vagus nerve stimulation remain intact, but a parathyroid suspect has not been identified, dissection should proceed similarly on the contralateral side. Normal parathyroid glands identified in the process should be preserved with an intact blood supply. Marking identified glands at the distal end with metal clips can aid in reidentification. If a lesion is still not identified, a cervical thymectomy may be performed. It is important to note that the traditional recommendation to perform a thyroid lobectomy on the higher probability side is relatively obsolete in the era of high-resolution ultrasonography. Instead, intrathyroidal candidates can be aspirated for PTH testing to determine candidacy before considering a lobectomy.

I Have Done All of the Above and I Still Cannot Find It

There are times when a surgeon anticipated a straightforward parathyroidectomy based on preoperative measures as described above, only to discover that the candidate lesion was a false positive or could not be identified. In rare instances, a patient may have a supernumerary parathyroid gland that is ectopic and dysfunctional. Furthermore, some parathyroid lesions are simply not accessible from the midline central neck approach. Mediastinal (intrathoracic) or retropharyngeal parathyroids may require a sternotomy or transoral approach for their removal. Anticipating these locations preoperatively is essential for patient counseling and surgical planning; otherwise, it is better for the surgeon to acknowledge an unsuccessful exploration, avoid morbidity, and terminate a parathyroidectomy procedure to enable further evaluation that could lead to successful revision surgery.

SUMMARY

Parathyroidectomy for PHPT, usually straightforward, can occasionally be anything but. A thorough preoperative preparation is the key to maximizing surgical success, minimizing morbidity, and avoiding the need for remedial evaluation and surgery.

CLINICS CARE POINTS

- Optimal preoperative preparation includes personally reviewing all images, relating candidate lesions to regional anatomy, and anticipating their location with respect to the nonvisible recurrent laryngeal nerves.
- The value of surgeon-performed ultrasonography, and examination of the entire neck, in the management of parathyroid disease cannot be overstated.
- Surgical adjuncts (serum intraoperative parathyroid hormone [PTH], PTH washout [from fine needle aspiration], autofluorescence, and selective venous sampling) can be helpful but are no substitute for meticulous surgical dissection.
- Lesions, especially superior parathyroids, are commonly deeper than expected, mandating dissection all the way to the prevertebral plane in many cases.

DISCLOSURE

Z.H. Fullerton has no disclosures. L.A. Orloff has participated on a Clinicians Advisory Board for Ascendis Pharma.

SUPPLEMENTARY DATA

Supplementary data related to this article can be found online at https://doi.org/10.1016/j.otc.2023.07.004.

REFERENCES

1. Hoang JK, Sung WK, Bahl M, et al. How to perform parathyroid 4D CT: tips and traps for technique and interpretation. Radiology 2014;270(1):15–24.
2. Hinson AM, Lee DR, Hobbs BA, et al. Preoperative 4D CT localization of nonlocalizing parathyroid adenomas by ultrasound and SPECT-CT. Otolaryngol Head Neck Surg 2015;153(5):775–8.
3. Steward DL, Danielson GP, Afman CE, et al. Parathyroid adenoma localization: surgeon-performed ultrasound versus sestamibi. Laryngoscope 2006;116(8):1380–4.
4. Devcic Z, Jeffrey RB, Kamaya A, et al. The elusive parathyroid adenoma: techniques for detection. Ultrasound Q 2013;29(3):179–87.
5. Battista RA, Noel JE, Orloff LA. Use of vascular clues to locate ectopic parathyroid glands and predict anatomic abnormalities. JAMA Otolaryngol Head Neck Surg 2021;147(2):211–3.
6. Cohen SM, Noel JE, Puccinelli CL, et al. Ultrasound identification of normal parathyroid glands. OTO Open 2021;5(4). 2473974X211052857.
7. Ruda JM, Hollenbeak CS, Stack BC. A systematic review of the diagnosis and treatment of primary hyperparathyroidism from 1995 to 2003. Otolaryngol Head Neck Surg 2005;132(3):359–72.
8. Pattou F, Huglo D, Proye C. Radionuclide scanning in parathyroid diseases. Br J Surg 1998;85(12):1605–16.
9. Mihai R, Gleeson F, Buley ID, et al. Negative imaging studies for primary hyperparathyroidism are unavoidable: correlation of sestamibi and high-resolution ultrasound scanning with histological analysis in 150 patients. World J Surg 2006;30(5):697–704.

10. Rodgers SE, Hunter GJ, Hamberg LM, et al. Improved preoperative planning for directed parathyroidectomy with 4-dimensional computed tomography. Surgery 2006;140(6):932–40 [discussion: 940-941].

11. Nguyen XV, Choudhury KR, Eastwood JD, et al. Incidental thyroid nodules on CT: evaluation of 2 risk-categorization methods for work-up of nodules. AJNR Am J Neuroradiol 2013;34(9):1812–7.

12. Bahl M, Muzaffar M, Vij G, et al. Prevalence of the polar vessel sign in parathyroid adenomas on the arterial phase of 4D CT. AJNR Am J Neuroradiol 2014;35(3): 578–81.

13. Madorin CA, Owen R, Coakley B, et al. Comparison of radiation exposure and cost between dynamic computed tomography and sestamibi scintigraphy for preoperative localization of parathyroid lesions. JAMA Surg 2013;148(6):500–3.

14. Memeh KO, Palacios JE, Khan R, et al. Pre-operative localization of parathyroid adenoma: performance of 4D MRI parathyroid protocol. Endocr Pract 2019;25(4): 361–5.

15. Nael K, Hur J, Bauer A, et al. Dynamic 4D MRI for characterization of parathyroid adenomas: multiparametric analysis. Am J Neuroradiol 2015;36(11):2147.

16. Grimaldi S, Young J, Kamenicky P, et al. Challenging pre-surgical localization of hyperfunctioning parathyroid glands in primary hyperparathyroidism: the added value of 18F-Fluorocholine PET/CT. Eur J Nucl Med Mol Imaging 2018;45(10): 1772–80.

17. Mathey C, Keyzer C, Blocklet D, et al. 18F-Fluorocholine PET/CT is more sensitive than 11C-Methionine PET/CT for the localization of hyperfunctioning parathyroid tissue in primary hyperparathyroidism. J Nucl Med 2022;63(5):785–91.

18. Norman J, Politz D, Browarsky I. Diagnostic aspiration of parathyroid adenomas causes severe fibrosis complicating surgery and final histologic diagnosis. Thyroid 2007;17(12):1251–5.

19. Ibraheem K, Toraih EA, Haddad AB, et al, Farag M, Randolph GW, Kandil E. Selective parathyroid venous sampling in primary hyperparathyroidism: a systematic review and meta-analysis. Laryngoscope 2018;128(11):2662–7.

20. Rajan S, Gracie D, Aspinall S. does surgeon volume impact morbidity following parathyroidectomy? A study of 16,140 parathyroidectomies from the UK registry of endocrine and thyroid surgery (UKRETS) database. World J Surg 2023;47(5): 1221–30.

21. Stuart H, Azab B, Roque OP, et al. Intraoperative parathormone monitoring to predict operative success in patients with normohormonal hyperparathyroidism. Can J Surg J Can Chir 2022;65(4):E468–73.

Autofluorescence of Parathyroid Glands

A Review of Methods of Parathyroid Gland Identification and Parathyroid Vascular Assessment

Amanda Silver Karcioglu, MD[a],*, Dana Hartl, MD[b],
David C. Shonka Jr, MD[c], Cristian M. Slough, MD[d],
Brendan C. Stack Jr, MD[d,e], Neil Tolley, MD FRCS DLO[f],
Amr H. Abdelhamid Ahmed, MBBCH, MMSc[g],
Gregory W. Randolph, MD[g,h]

KEYWORDS

- Near-infrared autofluorescence • Parathyroid gland • Thyroid surgery
- Hypoparathyroidism • Indocyanine green • Laser speckle

Continued

INTRODUCTION

Hypoparathyroidism, characterized by low calcium and absent or insufficient circulating parathyroid hormone (PTH), is most commonly a consequence of accidental injury or removal of parathyroid glands (PGs) during anterior neck surgery. Other

[a] Division of Otolaryngology–Head and Neck Surgery, Department of Surgery, NorthShore University HealthSystem, 9669 North Kenton Avenue, Suite 206, Skokie, IL 60076, USA; [b] Department of Surgery, Thyroid Surgery Unit, Gustave Roussy Cancer Campus and University Paris-Saclay, 114 rue Edouard Vaillant, Villejuif, Paris 94805, France; [c] Division of Head and Neck Surgery, Department of Otolaryngology–Head and Neck Surgery, University of Virginia, PO Box 800713, Charlottesville, VA 22903, USA; [d] Department of Otolaryngology–Head and Neck Surgery, Hawke's Bay Fallon Soldiers' Memorial Hospital, Te Whatu Ora Health New Zealand, 251 Orchard Road, Frimley, Hastings 4120, New Zealand; [e] Department of Otolaryngology– Head and Neck Surgery, Southern Illinois University School of Medicine, PO Box 19662, Springfield, IL 62794-9662, USA; [f] Department Otolaryngology–Head & Neck Surgery, St Mary's Hospital, Imperial College NHS Healthcare Trust, Praed Street, Paddington, London W2 1NY, UK; [g] Division of Thyroid and Parathyroid Endocrine Surgery, Department of Otolaryngology– Head and Neck Surgery, Massachusetts Eye and Ear Infirmary, Harvard Medical School, 243 Charles Street, Boston, MA 02114, USA; [h] Department of Surgery, Massachusetts General Hospital, Harvard Medical School, Boston, MA, USA

* Corresponding author. Thyroid and Parathyroid Endocrine Head and Neck Surgery, Division of Otolaryngology - Head and Neck Surgery, NorthShore University HealthSystem, 9669 North Kenton Avenue, Suite 206, Skokie, IL 60076.

E-mail address: akarcioglu@northshore.org

Otolaryngol Clin N Am 57 (2024) 139–154
https://doi.org/10.1016/j.otc.2023.07.011
0030-6665/24/© 2023 Elsevier Inc. All rights reserved.

oto.theclinics.com

Continued

KEY POINTS

- Postoperative hypoparathyroidism causes significant morbidity and even mortality.
- Emerging technologies using near-infrared-induced autofluorescence hold promise to improve surgical techniques to preserve parathyroid glands and possibly improve postoperative parathyroid gland function.
- Currently, probe-based and camera-based near-infrared autofluorescence systems are commercially available to assist in parathyroid gland identification during surgery, but alone do not provide the assessment of parathyroid gland perfusion or function.
- Near-infrared-induced autofluorescence combined with indocyanine green can inform parathyroid gland identification and subjective assessment of parathyroid gland perfusion.
- The application of near-infrared autofluorescence technologies in thyroid and parathyroid surgery is burgeoning, and additional work is needed to clarify the impact on relevant clinical outcomes.

causes are autoimmune or genetic.[1] The prevalence of hypoparathyroidism is estimated at 23 to 37 cases per 100,000.[2] Rates of permanent postoperative hypoparathyroidism are as high as 4% to 12.5%.[3–6]

Patients with permanent postoperative hypoparathyroidism show an increased incidence of renal failure, seizures, calcifications in the basal ganglia, decreased quality of life, and even mortality.[6–10] Postsurgical hypoparathyroidism is challenging to treat. Under treatment of pregnant patients can lead to premature delivery, intrauterine fetal hyperparathyroidism, and fetal death; over treatment can result in complications such as abortion, stillbirth, perinatal death, and neonatal tetany.[11–13] Postsurgical hypoparathyroidism in patients with a history of gastric bypass surgery poses a risk for recalcitrant hypocalcemia.[14–21] The management of hypoparathyroidism often includes a varied combination of activated vitamin D, calcium, magnesium, thiazides, phosphate binders, dietary and lifestyle changes, and recombinant human PTH.[1–3,10,22]

During surgery, the PGs small size, variable location, and similar appearance to surrounding tissues make reliable identification challenging. The assessment of adequate perfusion of PGs and prediction of postoperative function also pose challenges intraoperatively. As with intraoperative neural monitoring, technologies exist to help identify and potentially preserve PGs during thyroid surgery. Near-infrared autofluorescence (NIRAF) allows PGs to spontaneously emit light (autofluorescence) when exposed to a wavelength of 785 nm, allowing for differentiation both in vivo and ex vivo.[23–25] There is a learning curve to its successful implementation,[25,26] with possible false-negative and false-positive results (**Table 1**).[26] NIRAF is unable

Table 1
Potential false positives and false negatives

False Positives	False Negatives
• Brown fat or fibroadipose tissue	• Poor baseline calibration (probe-based system)
• Metastatic lymph nodules	• Inaccurate interpretation of qualitative data (camera-based system)
• Colloidal thyroid nodules	• Location of depth of PG in surgical field
	• Rare low-intensity normal PG
	• Secondary hyperparathyroidism
	• Deep-seated intrathyroidal parathyroid glands

to distinguish perfused from nonviable glands as autofluorescence persists even ex vivo.[24] Limitations to widespread adoption include the intraoperative learning curve, local availability, cost, standardization of its use, and lack of definitive data on improvement in clinical outcomes.

PARATHYROID GLAND IDENTIFICATION

PG preservation during thyroid surgery may be facilitated by early detection of the PGs, which may inform real-time surgical adjustments. Under near-infrared light, PGs exhibit autofluorescence, which may be used to improve PG identification. Current commercially available NIRAF systems include probe-based and camera- or image-based systems, and in 2018, The US Food and Drug Administration granted clearance a probe-based system (PTeye [Medtonic]) and a camera-based system (Fluobeam 800 and Fluobeam LX [Fluoptics]).[27]

PROBE-BASED SYSTEMS

Probe-based systems consist of a disposable sterile handheld probe, surgeon-activated foot pedal, and console with processor and visual display. The near-infrared laser and fluorescence spectrometer are integrated into the handheld probe and once activated provide a quantitative detection level, detection ratio, and an audible signal corresponding to the relative intensity of the fluorescent light compared with a baseline. The detection ratio is calculated by dividing the interrogated tissue detection level by the baseline level measured of the thyroid gland. The accurate establishment of the baseline with measurements of the normal thyroid tissue minimizes false positives and false negatives.

The benefits of the probe-based systems are the small-sized hand-held probe and the intuitive adoption for surgeons accustomed to using handheld recurrent laryngeal nerve monitoring systems.[28,29] The systems are easily portable and can be used in small surgical fields. The probe may be used repeatedly during surgery with minimal interruption of procedural flow and without dimming the room lights.

There is a learning curve however to proper utilization. Inaccurate calibration may yield possible false-positive and/or false-negative results (see **Table 1**). The probe should be used in a dry surgical field in direct contact with the interrogated tissue, thus the probe does not allow for a "field of view." The depth of penetration in ex vivo human tissues is limited to 0.4 to 5 mm.[30] The probe-based technology is not compatible with the use of indocyanine green (ICG).

The rate of parathyroid identification compared with visual identification alone is very high, with sensitivity greater than 95% (**Table 2**) and reported accuracy in intraoperative identification of PG(s) of 92% to 98%.[29,31,32] One prospective study found the probe system to have a higher sensitivity, specificity, and accuracy as compared with the camera-based technology and visual identification.[31] A meta-analysis however of 17 studies (1198 patients) found no significant difference in sensitivity or specificity between the two system types: probe-based systems had a higher negative predictive value and camera-based systems had a higher positive predictive value.[33] Clinical trials evaluating the effect of probe-based technologies to reduce postoperative hypoparathyroidism or inadvertent PG removal are underway.[34,35]

CAMERA-BASED SYSTEMS

Camera-based (image-based) systems consist of a handheld camera providing a near-infrared light source (typically 700–800 nm), a light detector optimized to near-infrared

Table 2
Summary of salient articles

Study	Design	Population	System	Number of Patients	Outcomes Measured	Results
RCT and Prospective Studies						
2023						
Lykke E, Eur Arch Oto-Rhino-Laryngol, 2023	Prospective randomized blinded 2 centers	TT Completion thyroidectomy	Camera	147 73 NIR 74 No NIR	HypoCa at 12 h HypoCa at 1 mo HypoCa at 3 mo Additional PG identified only with NIR	$P = .73$ $P = .50$ $P = .046$ (6.5% vs 11.8%) 9%
Huang, J Front Endocrinol, 2023	Prospective randomized	TT with bilateral neck dissection	Camera	100 NIRAF 50 Controls 50	Drop in PTH post-op day 1 and day 3 Number of PG identified Inadvertent resection	$P < .0001$ $P < .0001$ $P < .008$
Belcher RH, Laryngoscope, 2023	Prospective single-center	Pediatric Thyroidectomy Parathyroidectomy	Probe	19	Detection rate vs visual identification	95.8%
2022						
Wolf HW, Langenbecks, 2022	Prospective randomized single center	TT	Camera	60 NIRAF 30 Controls 30	Hypocalcemia PTH levels	NS Nonsignificant ($P = .058$)
Thomas G, Am J Surg, 2022	Prospective blinded single arm	TT Primary hyperparathyroidism	Probe	167	Sensitivity of probe vs surgeon eye or histopathology	92.7%

	Study design	Surgery	Device	N	Outcome	Results
2021						
Van Slycke S, Surg Innov, 2021	Prospective cohort	TT	Camera	1083 NIRAF 40 Controls 1043	All 4 PG identified Autotransplantation Temp HypoCa Perm HypoCa	35% (n = 14) vs 14.1% (n = 147) NS NIRAF 17.5% vs non-NIRAF 31.9% NIRAF 0% vs Non-NIRAF 3.1%
Papavramidis TS, Endocrine, 2021	Prospective randomized single-blind single center	TT	Camera	180 NIR 90 NONIR 90	Hypocalcemia Inadvertent resection	NS $P = .02$
Kiernan CM, J Sug Oncol, 2021	Prospective single center	Thyroidectomy Parathyroidectomy	Probe	83	Positive predictive value (PPV) Negative predictive value (NPV) Accuracy vs visual identification	93.0% 100% 94.3%
2020						
Benmiloud F, JAMA Surgery, 2020	Prospective randomized 3 centers	TT	Camera	241 NIRAF 121 Controls 120	Hypocalcemia day 1–2 Autotransplantation Inadvertent resection	OR 0.35 ($P = .017$) 3.3% vs 13.3% ($P = .009$) 2.5% vs 11.7% ($P = .006$)
2019						
Dip F, J Am Coll Surg, 2019	Camera randomized	TT	Camera	170 NIR 85 Controls 85	Number of PTH identified vs unaided eye Hypocalcemia	$P < .001$ $P = .005$
Thomas G, J Am Coll Surg, 2019	Prospective blinded single arm	TT Primary hyperparathyroidism	Camera + probe	20	Probe vs Camera vs observer	Sensitivity 97.0%- 90.9%-81.8% Specificity 84.2% - 73.7%-73.7% Accuracy 92.3%-84.6%- 78.8%

(continued on next page)

Table 2
(continued)

Study	Design	Population	System	Number of Patients	Outcomes Measured	Results
Meta-Analysis						
2022						
Kim DH, Langenbecks, 2022	Meta-analysis	Thyroidectomy Parathyroidectomy	Camera + probe	17 studies 1198 patients	Sensitivity Specificity NPV PPV	*Probe Camera P-value* .9788 .9634 .37 .9274 .9262 .973 .9790 .8851 (P = .0082) .9172 .9786 (P = .0486)
Lu W, J Invest Surg, 2022	Meta-analysis	Thyroidectomy	Camera + probe	8 studies 2889 patients	Temporary hypocalcemia Temporary hypoPTH Inadvertent resection Autotransplantation Permanent hypocalcemia	P < .0001 P = .0008 P < .0001 NS Nonsignificant
2021						
Wang B, Front Endocrinol, 2021	Meta-analysis	TT Primary hypoparathyroidism	Camera	7 studies 1480 patients	Inadvertent resection Autotransplantation Hypocalcemia day 1 Hypocalcemia 6 mo	RR 0.48 (P = .023) RR 0.39 (P = .2) RR 0.49 (P < .001) RR 0.34 (P = .238)
Weng YJ, Head Neck, 2021	Probe/camera meta-analysis	TT		6 studies 2180 patients	Temporary hypocalcemia Permanent hypocalcemia	P < .0001 P = .05
Other						
2023						
Barbieri D, Endocrine, 2023	Retrospective case-control	TT	Camera	NIRAF 67 Controls 67	Hypocalcemia PTH levels Oral calcium	P = .04 P = .01 P < .01

Year	Study	Design	Procedure	Device	N	Outcomes	P-value
2022	Domoslawski P, Int J Med Sci, 2022	Retrospective study	TT	Camera	65	Hypocalcemia	$P = .16$
						PTH levels	$P = .35$
2021	Kim DH, Thyroid, 2021	Retrospective	TT and central neck dissection	Camera	524 NIRAF 261 Controls 281	Temporary hypoPTH	$P = .001$
						Permanent hypoPTH	$P = .816$
						Hypocalcemia	NS
						Inadvertent resection	$P = .021$
2020	Kim YS, J Surg Oncol, 2020	Retrospective	TT	Camera	300 NIRAF 100 Controls 200	Temporary hypocalcemia	NS
						Permanent hypocalcemia	NS
						Inadvertent resection	$P = .039$
						Autotransplantation	$P = .562$
2019	DiMarco A, Ann R Coll Surg Eng, 2019	Prospective	Thyroidectomy	Camera	269 NIRAF 106 Controls 163	Inadvertent resection	NS
						Hypocalcemia	NS
						Hypoparathyroidism (at 1 d, 2 wk, 6 mo)	NS
2018	Benmiloud F, Surgery, 2018	Case control	TT	Camera	513 NIRAF 246 Controls 267	Hypocalcemia	$P < .001$
						Number of PTH identified	$P < .05$
						Autotransplantation	$P < .05$
						Inadvertent resection	NS

Abbreviations: NS, nonsignificant; TT, total thyroidectomy, thyroidectomy (including TT and thyroid lobectomy).

light (800–830 nm), a processor, and a visual display that shows the operating field on a grayscale screen to be assessed qualitatively. When combined with ICG for assessment of PG perfusion, a subjective 3-grade ICG score (0 = devascularized; 1 = moderately well vascularized; 2 = well vascularized) can be used[36]; however, other grading systems exist.[36–38] Once ICG has been administered, NIRAF can no longer be detected as the background ICG fluorescence is more intense than the NIRAF.

The camera is not in direct contact with the tissue and a "field of view" is provided. This offers the ability to scan the field. The depth of detection of unexposed parathyroids, however, ranges from 0.35 to 3.05 mm, with a mean depth of detection of 1.23 mm,[39] so deeper glands are not detected. For optimal efficacy, operating lights should be turned away from the field during interrogation; thus, the procedural flow may be interrupted. Camera-based systems cannot be used in smaller incisions. Importantly, the NIRAF image assessment remains qualitative.

Most of the parathyroid autofluorescence studies to date have used the camera-based system (see **Table 2**). In several studies, the camera was shown to enable the surgeon to detect more PGs than with the unaided eye and to reduce the rate of inadvertent resection of PGs. Some studies have shown a decrease in the rate of autotransplantation when using the device,[40] whereas two meta-analyses failed to find a significant difference.[41,42] The definition and rate of temporary hypocalcemia or hypoparathyroidism, however, varies among studies, with some studies failing to reach statistical significance. Three large meta-analyses found a significant reduction in the rate of temporary, but not permanent, postoperative hypoparathyroidism using the camera-based system for PG identification with NIRAF.

Both probe- and camera-based systems lack standardization and established norms. Importantly, neither system alone assesses perfusion or postoperative function of the PGs. **Table 3** provides a summary comparison of the probe- and camera-based systems.

VASCULAR ASSESSMENT OF PARATHYROID GLANDS

Intraoperative techniques to evaluate the vascular perfusion of the PGs during thyroid surgery have been studied with the goal of decreasing the rate of postoperative hypoparathyroidism.

INDOCYANINE GREEN FLUORESCENCE IMAGING

The most widely used surgical adjunct for determining the vascularity of PGs intraoperatively involves injection of ICG and near-infrared fluorescence (NIRF) imaging. ICG is an amphiphilic tricarbocyanine dye with a peak absorption spectrum of 780 to 805 nm and emission fluorescence of 820 to 835 nm. It is administered intravenously with a typical dose of 2.5 to 10 mg and fluorescence occurs 30 seconds to 2 minutes after injection, lasting up to 20 minutes.[25] Although repeated injections can be performed, the first set of images is typically the easiest to interpret due to less background ICG from prior injections. The first injection is most often performed after the thyroid has been removed, although alternative timing may be useful in certain situations.[25] ICG can be used with several different NIRAF camera-based systems.

The results of ICG combined with NIRF are mostly qualitative rather than quantitative. The most frequently used scoring systems assign each PG a score from 0 to 2 based on the degree of ICG fluorescence (0 = devascularized; 1 = moderately well vascularized; 2 = well vascularized).[36] Rarely, patients will have an allergic reaction to the injection, and ICG is not approved for use in pregnancy. Intraoperative bleeding may spill ICG into the surgical field confounding the results. It is important to note that

Table 3
Advantages and considerations of near-infrared autofluorescence systems

	Probe-Based Technology	Camera-Based Technology
Advantages	• Noninvasive • Semiquantitative • No need to dim the lights in the OR • Smaller, lighter, easier to handle • Easier to transport • Can be used in a small field during minimally invasive surgery • Cost	• Noninvasive • No contact with the patient • Visual mapping • Wide field of view • May show visually unidentified parathyroid glands • No need for baseline measures • Dissection can be performed with the camera images • Can be coupled with real-time color video • Can be coupled with ICG for angiography • Can be used for other surgical indications (ie, breast surgery, maxillofacial surgery)
Considerations	• PG must be exposed to the NIR light • Blood in the field may hinder detection • No anatomic images or spatial information provided • Can only test the tissue that is in contact with the probe (cannot show unidentified parathyroids • Only gives information in the small area tested • Probe must be sterile • Baseline measures must be accurate • False positives (ie, brown fat) • Cannot be used for ICG angiography	• PG must be exposed to the NIR light • Blood in the field may hinder detection • Must dim the lights in the OR • Needs a larger operating field • No quantification • Subjective interpretation • False-positive images • Accuracy may vary with camera distance and ambient light • More cumbersome to handle and transport • Cost

Note: Devices not yet validated for pediatric use.

NIRAF cannot be used after ICG NIRF imaging because the ICG obscures the autofluorescence from the PGs.

ICG NIRF imaging compares favorably with NIRAF for PG identification, but a limitation of ICG is lack of distinction from adjacent thyroid tissue.[43] ICG NIRF is therefore more often used to assess vascularity of PGs rather than to aid in their identification. Several studies have evaluated the utility of ICG for evaluating PG perfusion and subsequent postoperative parathyroid function after thyroid surgery.[25] An early study of 36 patients showed normal postoperative PTH levels when ICG showed at least one well-perfused PG.[37] One study sought to quantify ICG results by calculating the fluorescence intensity.[44] In this study of 70 patients undergoing total thyroidectomy, no patients with a greatest fluorescent light intensity greater than 150% developed postoperative hypocalcemia, whereas nine patients with greatest fluorescent light intensity less than 150% had hypocalcemia. A randomized controlled trial evaluated 196 patients who underwent ICG angiography during thyroid surgery.[36] In this study, 146 patients who had at least one well-vascularized PG on ICG were randomized to calcium supplementation and PTH testing versus no supplementation or testing and the no supplementation or PTH testing group was found to be non-inferior in the development of hypocalcemia. These studies support the ability of ICG NIRAF to predict normal postoperative PTH levels when at least one PG is well vascularized (ICG score 2).

Many of the studies of ICG are limited by lack of evaluation of all four PGs. It is difficult to determine an exact correlation of the ICG status of each PG with postoperative PTH levels. Some investigators have also raised concerns that ICG may overestimate PG devascularization.[45] Further studies evaluating cost-effectiveness and the utility of ICG use in the prevention of transient and permanent hypocalcemia are warranted.

LASER SPECKLE CONTRAST IMAGING

Laser speckle contrast imaging (LSCI) is a contrast-free angiography technique used to determine the viability of PGs intraoperatively.[46] This technique uses a laser to target tissue with coherent light. A detector collects the backscattered light and the dark and bright areas form a speckle pattern. Stationary tissue forms a constant speckle pattern, whereas movement in the tissue creates changes in the speckle pattern that can be quantified. A speckle contrast quantity is calculated where lower speckle contrast is associated with greater blood flow in the tissue.

Mannoh and colleagues reported the use of LSCI intraoperatively on 20 patients undergoing thyroidectomy (LSCI performed with noncommercially available equipment).[46] The average speckle contrast was compared with visual assessment of parathyroid perfusion by the surgeon, and PGs with decreased perfusion were found to have a higher average speckle contrast value. The same study validated the speckle contrast value on eight patients undergoing parathyroidectomy to mitigate the limitation of using a surgeon's visual assessment of gland viability as the gold standard. A follow-up study of 72 patients undergoing thyroidectomy compared the average speckle contrast value with PTH levels on postoperative day 1.[47] All PGs that identified during surgery were evaluated with LSCI and a speckle contrast value above 0.186 correlated with hypoparathyroidism postoperatively (87.5% sensitivity, 84.4% specificity). Imaging the identified glands (average 2.9 PGs per patient) added about 5 minutes to the total operative time. The advantages of LSCI include the quantifiable results that it does not interfere with NIRAF. A primary disadvantage is the lack of commercially available LSCI equipment. Future directions include the development of a handheld device that performs both LSCI and NIRAF seamlessly.

OTHER TECHNOLOGIES IN DEVELOPMENT FOR VASCULAR ASSESSMENT

Several other label-free parathyroid assessment tools are in earlier stages of evaluation and development but have exiting potential future applications. Optical coherence tomography (OCT) uses near-infrared light interferometry to generate two-dimensional images similar to ultrasound but with 10 times the resolution. Although ex vivo studies have demonstrated high sensitivity in differentiating parathyroid tissue from thyroid, lymph nodes, and fat,[48] similar results have been lacking in vivo, particularly when attempting to distinguish parathyroid tissue from lymph nodes.[49] However, the resolution is such that OCT may have a future role in defining the microvascularity supplying PGs in real time to aid in the preservation of perfusion.

NIRAF can be affected by intensity artifacts and tissues with similarly high NIRAF can cause false positives. Fluorescence lifetime imaging microscopy is less prone to intensity-related artifacts but its use has been limited thus far by long scanning times and shallow depth of view.[50]

Dynamic optical contrast imaging has been shown to reliably identify parathyroid tissue in ex vivo samples with a shorter acquisition time (<2 minutes), and current work is underway to further evaluate this tool in the clinical setting.[51]

Raman spectroscopy is a powerful, label-free optical analytical tool for evaluating the biochemical composition of biological tissues. Clinical applications have also been limited by time-consuming measurements, but acquisition time is expected to diminish with technological advancements. A recent study has demonstrated the ability of Raman spectroscopy (RS) to distinguish normal from abnormal parathyroid tissue in hyperparathyroidism.[52]

CLINICAL APPLICATION OF NEAR-INFRARED-INDUCED AUTOFLUORESCENCE

NIRAF has been successfully applied in other facets of surgery such as the detection of colorectal adenomas in high-risk patients with familial colorectal cancer syndromes.[53] Paras and colleagues (Vanderbilt University) discovered the autofluorescent properties of the PG and its applicability in thyroid and parathyroid surgery.[23,54] Further work showed its clinical utility and reliability in the detection of the PG intraoperatively.[55,56] NIRAF has been shown to be useful for the identification of the PG during thyroid surgery across a range of thyroid disease states including toxic and nontoxic nodular goiters, Hashimoto's thyroiditis, Follicular and Hurthle cell thyroid adenomas, Medullary thyroid carcinoma, Graves' disease, and well-differentiated thyroid carcinoma.

McWade and colleagues investigated 264 PGs (137 patients) using NIRAF to successfully identify 97% PGs intraoperatively.[55] Studies by De Leeuw[24] and colleagues and Liu[57] showed that NIRAF identification correlates with histologic verification. In Liu's study, autofluorescence had a 100% sensitivity for gland identification and a 90% ability to differentiate parathyroid tissue from surrounding tissue with a 95% positive predictive value.[57] Ladurner and colleagues in their experience with NIRAF over 5 years found that autofluorescence was able to identify 87% of PGs.[58]

NIRAF technology also allows potentially earlier identification of PGs during surgery to enable the surgeon to better understand the individual anatomy and facilitate preservation of gland perfusion by adjusting surgical technique in real time. This may be especially useful in thyroidectomy with concurrent central neck dissection when the PGs are at particular high risk of injury.[58]

The incidence of inadvertent parathyroidectomy during thyroid surgery has been reported to be between 8% and 22%.[59–62] Owing to a half-life of 152 hours ex vivo of the gland autofluorescence, this technology may be used to identify glands inadvertently removed on the thyroid specimen[63] especially in large goiters, by meticulously inspecting the surface of the thyroid gland for parathyroid tissue before formalin fixation which then may be autotransplanted. NIRAF has been shown to increase the rate of PG detection during surgery compared with the unaided eye, resulting in a decreased rate of autotransplantation and postoperative hypocalcemia.[64,65] A recent meta-analysis found NIRAF facilitated PG identification and reduced both the rate of autotransplantation and inadvertent resection.[66] The benefit of NIRAF may be during the immediate postoperative period as opposed to a decrease in permanent hypoparathyroidism rate.[66] NIRAF is particularly useful in reoperative surgery where identification and preservation of the remaining glands can be challenging.[67]

NIRAF is not only useful during thyroid surgery but has application in parathyroid surgery. It can aid the identification of abnormal and ectopic glands (allowing for the limitations in depth of penetration).[30,39] The technology can assist also in distinguishing parathyroid tissue from fat, a thyroid nodule, and lymph nodes.[67] This can be particularly useful when a gland is well localized and a focused or minimally invasive approach is being considered. In addition, if bilateral exploration is planned, it may help localize all four glands for assessment and can help identify and confirm (without the need for frozen section) an ectopic parathyroid when its location is outside the normal operative field.[67] When intraoperative PTH assays fail to normalize following suspected adenoma resection NIRAF can also be used to assess other sites such as the carotid sheath.

Some NIRAF systems use endoscopes. This technology has application with endoscopic approaches to both thyroid and parathyroid surgery, such as in thoracoscopic techniques thereby widening its applicability in endocrine surgery.[58,68]

SUMMARY

The use of NIRAF in thyroid and parathyroid surgery has shown promising results in aiding surgeons in identifying and preserving PGs during central neck surgery. By providing real-time visualization of tissue autofluorescence, it permits, without frozen section, a more accurate identification of the PGs, differentiating the glands from surrounding tissues and potentially reducing the risk of unintentional removal or damage. When accidently removed, NIRAF may facilitate ex vivo identification and reimplantation. Although further studies are needed to validate the technology with respect to long-term clinical outcomes, at present the technology seems to reduce the incidence of temporary hypoparathyroidism. The technology has the potential to improve surgical outcomes and reduce postoperative complications for patients undergoing thyroid and parathyroid surgery.

DISCLOSURE

Dr G.W. Randolph has received research grants (no personal fees) from Eisai, United States, Medtronic, and Fluoptics. Dr G.W. Randolph is the program director of the Mass. Eye & Ear Infirmary Endocrine Surgery Clinical Fellowship, which receives partial funding from Medtronic. Dr G.W. Randolph is the President of the International Thyroid Oncology Group (ITOG) and the World Congress on Thyroid Cancer (WCTC), is Chair of the Administrative Division of the American Head and Neck Society (AHNS), and is the American College of Surgeons (ACS) Otolaryngology Governor. All other authors have no conflicts to disclose.

REFERENCES

1. Mannstadt M, Bilezikian JP, Thakker RV, et al. Hypoparathyroidism. Nat Rev Dis Primer 2017;3:17055.

 2. Brandi ML, Bilezikian JP, Shoback D, et al. Management of Hypoparathyroidism: Summary Statement and Guidelines. J Clin Endocrinol Metab 2016;101(6): 2273–83.
 3. Annebäck M, Hedberg J, Almquist M, et al. Risk of Permanent Hypoparathyroidism After Total Thyroidectomy for Benign Disease: A Nationwide Population-based Cohort Study From Sweden. Ann Surg 2021;274(6):e1202–8.
 4. Stack BC, Twining C, Rastatter J, et al. Consensus statement by the American Association of Clinical Endocrinology (AACE) and the American Head and Neck Society Endocrine Surgery Section (AHNS-ES) on Pediatric Benign and Malignant Thyroid Surgery. Head Neck 2021;43(4):1027–42.
 5. Orloff LA, Wiseman SM, Bernet VJ, et al. American Thyroid Association Statement on Postoperative Hypoparathyroidism: Diagnosis, Prevention, and Management in Adults. Thyroid Off J Am Thyroid Assoc 2018;28(7):830–41.
 6. Almquist M, Ivarsson K, Nordenström E, et al. Mortality in patients with permanent hypoparathyroidism after total thyroidectomy. Br J Surg 2018;105(10):1313–8.
 7. Underbjerg L, Sikjaer T, Mosekilde L, et al. Cardiovascular and renal complications to postsurgical hypoparathyroidism: a Danish nationwide controlled historic follow-up study. J Bone Miner Res Off J Am Soc Bone Miner Res 2013;28(11): 2277–85.
 8. Bergenfelz A, Nordenström E, Almquist M. Morbidity in patients with permanent hypoparathyroidism after total thyroidectomy. Surgery 2020;167(1):124–8.
 9. Mitchell DM, Regan S, Cooley MR, et al. Long-term follow-up of patients with hypoparathyroidism. J Clin Endocrinol Metab 2012;97(12):4507–14.
10. Büttner M, Musholt TJ, Singer S. Quality of life in patients with hypoparathyroidism receiving standard treatment: a systematic review. Endocrine 2017;58(1): 14–20.
11. Khan AA, Clarke B, Rejnmark L, et al. MANAGEMENT OF ENDOCRINE DISEASE: Hypoparathyroidism in pregnancy: review and evidence-based recommendations for management. Eur J Endocrinol 2019;180(2):R37–44.
12. Hartogsohn EAR, Khan AA, Kjaersulf LU, et al. Changes in treatment needs of hypoparathyroidism during pregnancy and lactation: A case series. Clin Endocrinol 2020;93(3):261–8.
13. Lebrun B, De Block C, Jacquemyn Y. Hypocalcemia After Thyroidectomy and Parathyroidectomy in a Pregnant Woman. Endocrinology 2020;161(7).
14. Goldenberg D, Ferris RL, Shindo ML, et al. Thyroidectomy in patients who have undergone gastric bypass surgery. Head Neck 2018;40(6):1237–44.
15. Allo Miguel G, García Fernández E, Martínez Díaz-Guerra G, et al. Recalcitrant hypocalcaemia in a patient with post-thyroidectomy hypoparathyroidism and Roux-en-Y gastric bypass. Obes Res Clin Pract 2016;10(3):344–7.
16. Panazzolo DG, Braga TG, Bergamim A, et al. Hypoparathyroidism after Roux-en-Y gastric bypass–a challenge for clinical management: a case report. J Med Case Reports 2014;8:357.
17. Pietras SM, Holick MF. Refractory hypocalcemia following near-total thyroidectomy in a patient with a prior Roux-en-Y gastric bypass. Obes Surg 2009;19(4): 524–6.
18. Campos GM, Ziemelis M, Paparodis R, et al. Laparoscopic reversal of Roux-en-Y gastric bypass: technique and utility for treatment of endocrine complications. Surg Obes Relat Dis Off J Am Soc Bariatr Surg 2014;10(1):36–43.
19. Zaarour M, Zaharia R, Bretault M, et al. Laparoscopic Revision of Bariatric Surgeries in Two Patients with Severe Resistant Hypocalcemia After Endocrine Cervical Surgery. Obes Surg 2020;30(4):1616–20.

20. Corbeels K, Steenackers N, Lannoo M, et al. Reversal of Roux-en-Y Gastric Bypass Fails to Facilitate the Management of Recalcitrant Hypocalcaemia Caused by Primary Hypoparathyroidism. Obes Surg 2020. https://doi.org/10.1007/s11695-020-04903-8.

21. Droeser RA, Ottosson J, Muth A, et al. Hypoparathyroidism after total thyroidectomy in patients with previous gastric bypass. Langenbeck's Arch Surg 2017; 402(2):273–80.

22. Mannstadt M, Clarke BL, Vokes T, et al. Efficacy and safety of recombinant human parathyroid hormone (1-84) in hypoparathyroidism (REPLACE): a double-blind, placebo-controlled, randomised, phase 3 study. Lancet Diabetes Endocrinol 2013;1(4):275–83.

23. Paras C, Keller M, White L, et al. Near-infrared autofluorescence for the detection of parathyroid glands. J Biomed Opt 2011;16(6):067012.

24. De Leeuw F, Breuskin I, Abbaci M, et al. Intraoperative Near-infrared Imaging for Parathyroid Gland Identification by Auto-fluorescence: A Feasibility Study. World J Surg 2016;40(9):2131–8.

25. Silver Karcioglu AL, Triponez F, Solórzano CC, et al. Emerging Imaging Technologies for Parathyroid Gland Identification and Vascular Assessment in Thyroid Surgery: A Review From the American Head and Neck Society Endocrine Surgery Section. JAMA Otolaryngol Head Neck Surg 2023;149(3):253–60.

26. Hartl D, Obongo R, Guerlain J, et al. Intraoperative Parathyroid Gland Identification Using Autofluorescence: Pearls and Pitfalls. World J Surg Surg Res 2019;2: 1166.

27. FDA press release. Published November 2, 2018 Available at: https://www.fda.gov/news-events/press-announcements/fda-permits-marketing-two-devices-detect-parathyroid-tissue-real-time-during-surgery. Accessed April 22, 2023.

28. Solórzano CC, Thomas G, Baregamian N, et al. Detecting the Near Infrared Autofluorescence of the Human Parathyroid: Hype or Opportunity? Ann Surg 2019.

29. Thomas G, McWade MA, Nguyen JQ, et al. Innovative surgical guidance for label-free real-time parathyroid identification. Surgery 2019;165(1):114–23.

30. Stolik S, Delgado JA, Pérez A, et al. Measurement of the penetration depths of red and near infrared light in human "ex vivo" tissues. J Photochem Photobiol, B 2000;57(2–3):90–3.

31. Thomas G, Squires MH, Metcalf T, et al. Imaging or Fiber Probe-Based Approach? Assessing Different Methods to Detect Near Infrared Autofluorescence for Intraoperative Parathyroid Identification. J Am Coll Surg 2019;229(6): 596–608.e3.

32. Kiernan CM, Thomas G, Baregamian N, et al. Initial clinical experiences using the intraoperative probe-based parathyroid autofluorescence identification system—PTeye™ during thyroid and parathyroid procedures. J Surg Oncol 2021;124(3): 271–81.

33. Kim DH, Lee S, Jung J, et al. Near-infrared autofluorescence-based parathyroid glands identification in the thyroidectomy or parathyroidectomy: a systematic review and meta-analysis. Langenbeck's Arch Surg 2022;407(2):491–9.

34. Evaluating Impact of NIRAF Detection for Identifying Parathyroid Glands During Parathyroidectomy (NIRAF) https://clinicaltrials.gov/ct2/show/NCT04299425). Accessed April 22, 2023.

35. Assessing Benefits of NIRAF Detection for Identifying Parathyroid Glands During Total Thyroidectomy. (NIRAF). Accessed April 22, 2023. https://clinicaltrials.gov/ct2/show/NCT04281875. Accessed April 22, 2023.

36. Vidal Fortuny J, Sadowski SM, Belfontali V, et al. Randomized clinical trial of intra-operative parathyroid gland angiography with indocyanine green fluorescence predicting parathyroid function after thyroid surgery. Br J Surg 2018;105(4): 350–7.

37. Vidal Fortuny J, Belfontali V, Sadowski SM, et al. Parathyroid gland angiography with indocyanine green fluorescence to predict parathyroid function after thyroid surgery. Br J Surg 2016;103(5):537–43.

38. Zaidi N, Bucak E, Yazici P, et al. The feasibility of indocyanine green fluorescence imaging for identifying and assessing the perfusion of parathyroid glands during total thyroidectomy. J Surg Oncol 2016;113(7):775–8.

39. Han YS, Kim Y, Lee HS, et al. Detectable depth of unexposed parathyroid glands using near-infrared autofluorescence imaging in thyroid surgery. Front Endocrinol 2023;14:1170751.

40. Benmiloud F, Godiris-Petit G, Gras R, et al. Association of Autofluorescence-Based Detection of the Parathyroid Glands During Total Thyroidectomy With Post-operative Hypocalcemia Risk: Results of the PARAFLUO Multicenter Randomized Clinical Trial. JAMA Surg 2020;155(2):106–12.

41. Wang B, Zhu CR, Liu H, et al. The Accuracy of Near Infrared Autofluorescence in Identifying Parathyroid Gland During Thyroid and Parathyroid Surgery: A Meta-Analysis. Front Endocrinol 2021;12:701253.

42. Lu W, Chen Q, Zhang P, et al. Near-Infrared Autofluorescence Imaging in Thyroid Surgery: A Systematic Review and Meta-Analysis. J Investig Surg Off J Acad Surg Res 2022;35(9):1723–32.

43. Kahramangil B, Berber E. Comparison of indocyanine green fluorescence and parathyroid autofluorescence imaging in the identification of parathyroid glands during thyroidectomy. Gland Surg 2017;6(6):644–8.

44. Lang BHH, Wong CKH, Hung HT, et al. Indocyanine green fluorescence angiography for quantitative evaluation of in situ parathyroid gland perfusion and function after total thyroidectomy. Surgery 2017;161(1):87–95.

45. Razavi AC, Ibraheem K, Haddad A, et al. Efficacy of indocyanine green fluorescence in predicting parathyroid vascularization during thyroid surgery. Head Neck 2019;41(9):3276–81.

46. Mannoh EA, Thomas G, Solórzano CC, et al. Intraoperative Assessment of Parathyroid Viability using Laser Speckle Contrast Imaging. Sci Rep 2017;7(1):14798.

47. Mannoh EA, Thomas G, Baregamian N, et al. Assessing Intraoperative Laser Speckle Contrast Imaging of Parathyroid Glands in Relation to Total Thyroidectomy Patient Outcomes. Thyroid Off J Am Thyroid Assoc 2021;31(10):1558–65.

48. Conti de Freitas LC, Phelan E, Liu L, et al. Optical coherence tomography imaging during thyroid and parathyroid surgery: a novel system of tissue identification and differentiation to obviate tissue resection and frozen section. Head Neck 2014;36(9):1329–34.

49. Sommerey S, Al Arabi N, Ladurner R, et al. Intraoperative optical coherence tomography imaging to identify parathyroid glands. Surg Endosc 2015;29(9): 2698–704.

50. Hu Y, Han AY, Huang S, et al. A Tool to Locate Parathyroid Glands Using Dynamic Optical Contrast Imaging. Laryngoscope 2021;131(10):2391–7.

51. Kim IA, Taylor ZD, Cheng H, et al. Dynamic optical contrast imaging. Otolaryngol Head Neck Surg 2017;156(3):480–3.

52. Palermo A, Fosca M, Tabacco G, et al. Raman Spectroscopy Applied to Parathyroid Tissues: A New Diagnostic Tool to Discriminate Normal Tissue from Adenoma. Anal Chem 2018;90(1):847–54.

53. Ramsoekh D, Haringsma J, Poley JW, et al. A back-to-back comparison of white light video endoscopy with autofluorescence endoscopy for adenoma detection in high-risk subjects. Gut 2010;59(6):785–93.

54. McWade MA, Paras C, White LM, et al. Label-free Intraoperative Parathyroid Localization With Near-Infrared Autofluorescence Imaging. J Clin Endocrinol Metab 2014;99(12):4574–80.

55. McWade MA, Sanders ME, Broome JT, et al. Establishing the clinical utility of autofluorescence spectroscopy for parathyroid detection. Surgery 2016;159(1):193–203.

56. McWade MA, Paras C, White LM, et al. A novel optical approach to intraoperative detection of parathyroid glands. Surgery 2013;154(6):1371–7.

57. Liu J, Wang X, Wang R, et al. Near-infrared auto-fluorescence spectroscopy combining with Fisher's linear discriminant analysis improves intraoperative real-time identification of normal parathyroid in thyroidectomy. BMC Surg 2020;20(1):4.

58. Ladurner R, Lerchenberger M, Al Arabi N, et al. Parathyroid Autofluorescence-How Does It Affect Parathyroid and Thyroid Surgery? A 5 Year Experience. Mol Basel Switz 2019;24(14):2560.

59. Lee NJ, Blakey JD, Bhuta S, et al. Unintentional Parathyroidectomy During Thyroidectomy. Laryngoscope 1999;109(8):1238–40.

60. Sasson AR, Pingpank JF Jr, Wetherington RW, et al. Incidental Parathyroidectomy During Thyroid Surgery Does Not Cause Transient Symptomatic Hypocalcemia. Arch Otolaryngol Neck Surg 2001;127(3):304.

61. Sakorafas GH, Stafyla V, Bramis C, et al. Incidental Parathyroidectomy during Thyroid Surgery: An Underappreciated Complication of Thyroidectomy. World J Surg 2005;29(12):1539–43.

62. Barrios L, Shafqat I, Alam U, et al. Incidental parathyroidectomy in thyroidectomy and central neck dissection. Surgery 2021;169(5):1145–51.

63. McWade M. Development of an intraoperative tool to detect parathyroid gland autofluorescence. Available at: http://setdlibraryvanderbilteduavailableetd-041 52016-131447unrestrictedMcWadepdf. 2016.

64. Benmiloud F, Rebaudet S, Varoquaux A, et al. Impact of autofluorescence-based identification of parathyroids during total thyroidectomy on postoperative hypocalcemia: a before and after controlled study. Surgery 2018;163(1):23–30.

65. Dip F, Falco J, Verna S, et al. Randomized Controlled Trial Comparing White Light with Near-Infrared Autofluorescence for Parathyroid Gland Identification During Total Thyroidectomy. J Am Coll Surg 2019;228(5):744–51.

66. Wang B, Zhu CR, Liu H, et al. The Ability of Near-Infrared Autofluorescence to Protect Parathyroid Gland Function During Thyroid Surgery: A Meta-Analysis. Front Endocrinol 2021;12:714691.

67. Solórzano CC, Thomas G, Berber E, et al. Current state of intraoperative use of near infrared fluorescence for parathyroid identification and preservation. Surgery 2021;169(4):868–78.

68. Thammineedi SR, Saksena AR, Nusrath S, et al. Fluorescence-guided cancer surgery—A new paradigm. J Surg Oncol 2021;123(8):1679–98.

Future Directions in the Treatment of Thyroid and Parathyroid Disease

Pia Pace-Asciak, MASc, MD, FRCSC[a],*, Ralph P. Tufano, MD, MBA[b]

KEYWORDS

- Remote access robotic surgery • Parathyroid and thyroid disease • Thermal ablation
- Parathyroid autofluorescence • Artificial intelligence • Diagnostics

KEY POINTS

- In remote access surgery, future research is directed toward improving the ergonomics of robotic surgery, haptic feedback, as well as the incorporation of augmented reality.
- Optical imaging techniques, including near-infrared autofluorescence and indocyanine green-based fluorescence of the parathyroid glands, are innovative approaches that may play an increasingly important role in thyroid and parathyroid surgery.
- A range of ablative techniques now offer alternative treatments options to patients for benign nonfunctioning and functioning thyroid nodules, low risk well-differentiated thyroid cancer, as well as primary hyperparathyroidism.
- Artificial intelligence is being incorporated into diagnostics for improving the efficacy and workflow in thyroid and parathyroid diseases.

INTRODUCTION

Medicine is in the midst of a technological revolution where conventional practices in health care are being challenged. The fourth wave, or the digital revolution, is building on the third wave, known as the industrial revolution and finding ways to improve the efficiency and safety in patient care. Various fields of medicine are becoming more personalized and tailored to meet differing patient needs. During the past 2 decades, there have been new developments for managing thyroid and parathyroid disease in a less-invasive way both surgically and nonsurgically. These technological advancements have progressed toward improving outcomes, decreasing complications, and mainly, enhancing patients' quality of life.

[a] Department of Otolaryngology–Head and Neck Surgery, Temerty Faculty of Medicine, University of Toronto, Toronto, Canada; [b] Sarasota Memorial Health Care System Multidisciplinary Thyroid and Parathyroid Center, Sarasota, FL, USA
* Corresponding author.
E-mail addresses: piapaceasciak@gmail.com; Pia.Pace-Asciak@unityhealth.to

Otolaryngol Clin N Am 57 (2024) 155–170
https://doi.org/10.1016/j.otc.2023.07.013
0030-6665/24/© 2023 Elsevier Inc. All rights reserved.

Herein, we review the surgical and nonsurgical advancements for managing thyroid and parathyroid disease in remote access thyroid and parathyroid surgery. Specifically, we discuss the use of autofluorescence detection technology of the parathyroid glands to help mitigate hypocalcemia as well as the use of thermal ablation to target thyroid nodules directly. We also explore the possible influence of artificial intelligence (AI) on diagnostic approaches that are part of every workup in endocrinology to triage or improve surgical outcomes. In discussing the shortcomings of each advancement, we look at areas for targeting future research.

Surgical Advancements for the Management of Thyroid and Parathyroid Disease

Remote access Thyroidectomy and Parathyroidectomy

The desire to avoid having a neck scar has led to the development of endoscopic and remote access techniques for removing the thyroid. The impetus toward this movement is mainly cultural, particularly in Asian countries where scarring is viewed as an anathema. By comparison, North America has been slower to adopt remote access techniques due to the costly equipment and steep learning curve associated with remote access thyroid surgery. Regardless, robotic thyroid surgery has been adopted in several centers in the United States, and was introduced 2 decades ago to provide technical improvements to standard endoscopic thyroid surgery.[1]

Several meta-analysis studies have reported improved quality of life, safety, and surgical completeness when robotic thyroid surgery is compared with conventional open surgery for benign disease and low-risk thyroid cancer.[2–6] Various remote access approaches exist, which include the gasless transaxillary approach, bilateral axillo-breast approach, retroauricular approach, transoral vestibular approach, and others.[7–9] Even though each technique shares the common goal of avoiding a visible central neck incision, individual differences exist between techniques and some require extensive soft tissue dissection to gain adequate exposure of the thyroid. The transoral vestibular approach has gained favor for its direct access to the thyroid, parathyroid glands, and central neck from an incision in the mandibular gingivobuccal sulcus without leaving a cutaneous scar.[10–15] Regardless of where the incision is placed, robotic surgery represents a significant advancement in that it offers a three-dimensional magnified view, tremor filtering system, and flexible endo-wrist movement for access to tissue in smaller cavities.[12]

As with any new technology, there are shortcomings, particularly with navigating bulky robotic equipment in a small space such as the head and neck region. Since the introduction of the original robotic system, there have been several developments made to overcome its initial limitations. The transoral vestibular approach was first described with the use of the DaVinci robot (Intuitive Surgical, Sunnyvale, CA) and then adapted for an endoscopic approach, which was found to be more efficient, less cumbersome, and less costly.[16] As newer robotic systems are being developed, miniaturized robotic arms are being incorporated to allow for smaller endoscopes and instruments that are easy to navigate, making it a viable option in the pediatric population as well as for accessing smaller cavities in the head and neck.[17,18] The development of nanorobotics as well as autonomous surgical robots are other areas under active development.

Open thyroid surgery allows the surgeon to palpate the nodule of interest as well as nearby structures to identify hidden tissue and/or lymph nodes, whereas robotic approaches are limited in this respect. The lack of tactile feedback or the ability to detect the amount of force being applied to tissue during dissection can lead to complications. Improving the precision and accuracy of haptic feedback to avoid relying on visual cues alone is an area of active research.[19] Restoring the sense of touch and the ability to characterize the tissue being dissected may decrease the number of errors during blunt dissection and reduce the frequency of intraoperative tissue damage.[20] This shift from conventional approaches also introduces the need for simulators in endocrine head and neck surgery during residency and/or while in practice to become comfortable with remote access approaches, reduce the learning curve, and improve trouble shooting.[21]

Other areas of innovation stem from the integration of image guidance for navigating critical structures similar to the developments seen with endoscopic sinus surgery. Augmented reality (AR) is being used in surgery to enable virtual images of the organs to be overlaid onto the actual organs during surgery.[22–24] Lee and colleagues developed a vision-based tracking system for AR and evaluated whether this system enabled surgeons to locate the recurrent laryngeal nerve (RLN) during robotic thyroid surgery.[23] Using CT scan images, an AR image was constructed of the trachea and common carotid artery and overlaid on the physical structures once surgically exposed. Reasonable accuracy was achieved where a mean distance between the RLN AR image and the actual RLN was a couple of millimeters (1.9 ± 1.5 mm, range 0.5–3.7). As this type of technology evolves, AR may help enhance surgical safety, aid surgeons in finding hidden structures, and supplement the lack of tactile feedback found in robotic surgery.

Around the world, the list of indications for robotic thyroid and parathyroid surgery continue to expand. Generally, benign and low-risk thyroid cancers are acceptable candidates for robotic thyroid surgery.[2,25–27] Newer studies are expanding the indications to include resection of central and lateral neck disease.[25,28,29] Wang and colleagues, compared 80 patients who underwent central neck dissection (CND) using Transoral endoscopic thyroidectomy vestibular approach (TOETVA) to patients undergoing the open approach and found a similar number of positive lymph nodes dissected, complications, and time to complete the surgery.[25] Kim and colleagues, retrospectively, reviewed 476 patients that underwent robotic transaxillary lateral neck dissection (bilateral in 30 patients and unilateral 446 patients) for metastatic lateral neck disease from their papillary thyroid cancer.[28] Effective and safe surgery was demonstrated with only 5 cases of recurrence after their surgery. Future studies will continue to push the boundaries, and will likely expand the indications for remote access surgery.

Near-Infrared Autofluorescence of the Parathyroid Glands

Thyroid and parathyroid surgery is a common and safe surgery with very few complications. However, permanent postoperative hypocalcemia (greater than 6 months) can have a significant influence on the quality of life of patients and require a lifetime of calcium replacement. Inadvertent removal of a parathyroid gland or devascularization of the gland can occur despite careful dissection, even in experienced hands. If this occurs intraoperatively, the standard approach is to autotransplant morselized parathyroid fragments into the sternocleidomastoid muscle.[30] However, if the parathyroid gland is intrathyroidal or hidden, accidental removal can occur. The incidental finding of a parathyroid gland within the resected thyroid specimen is often noted by the pathologist in up to 22% of thyroidectomies.[31] Typically, the rate of permanent hypoparathyroidism is reported to occur in 1% to 4% of patients after total thyroidectomy.[32] However, more recent national registry studies report rates more than 10%. In an attempt to improve the rates of hypocalcemia postsurgery, technological advancements have been developed to assist surgeons in the intraoperative localization of these small glands.

One of the great discoveries in the early 1800s by Sir David Brewster is that parathyroid tissue contains intrinsic "fluorophores" causing the tissue to fluoresce.[33]

Subsequently, George Gabriel Stokes coined the phenomenon whereby the wavelength of light emitted by a given tissue differs from that of the exciting light, known as the "Stokes shift."[33] The term autofluorescence describes the emission of light by a naturally occurring fluorophore, which occurs when excited by an external light source of a specific wavelength (infrared spectrum).[34] During autofluorescence of the glands, parathyroid tissue is differentiated from the normal surrounding tissue without the need for any labeling or contrast agents. This confirms the location of the parathyroid glands intraoperatively and creates a so-called optical biopsy in the surgical field, without actually requiring removal of the tissue for frozen section. As a result, parathyroid autofluorescence has emerged as an intraoperative technique to help with the identification of parathyroid glands and to supplement direct visualization during thyroidectomy and parathyroidectomy. The use of near-infrared autofluorescence (NIRAF) has been reported to identify 76.3% to 100% of parathyroid glands intraoperatively and thus has been reported to reduce the incidence of postoperative hypocalcemia.[35]

Different technological approaches for detecting parathyroid glands via autofluorescence have been developed; camera-based and probe-based approaches have been approved by the US Food and Drug Administration.[36] The camera-based approach provides spatial visualization of the parathyroid glands without tissue contact compared with the probe-based system, which provides visual and auditory quantification once the parathyroid gland is isolated and the tissue is in contact with the probe. In a meta-analysis of 17 studies with 1198 patients, both the image-based and probe-based technology showed high diagnostic accuracy.[37] The probe-based method showed an improved diagnostic accuracy when the 2 NIRAF systems were compared in the same subject.[37,38]

NIRAF is helpful for identifying parathyroid tissue; however, identifying the parathyroid glands intraoperatively does not always equate to normal biochemical function or viability of the gland.[39] To assess the vascularity of the gland and thus predict the viability and function of the parathyroid gland, an extrinsic fluorescent contrast dye such as indocyanine green (ICG) can be added. This fluorescence (rather than autofluorescence) imaging, as an exogenous agent, is acting as the fluorophore. Generally, the injection of ICG is quick and allows for the arterial and venous drainage of the parathyroid gland to be observed using a NIRAF device over the exposed gland.[40] From this point, decisions can be made whether to autotransplant a potentially nonviable gland. In a randomized control trial of 180 patients, Yin and colleagues found a significant reduction in postoperative temporary hypoparathyroidism in the NIRAF/ICG group compared with the control group undergoing total thyroidectomy with unilateral or bilateral CND for papillary thyroid cancer (27.8% vs 43.3%, $P = .029$).[41] Benmiloud and colleagues found in their randomized clinical trial of 241 patients undergoing total thyroidectomy that NIRAF helped lower temporary postoperative hypocalcemia from 22% to 9% and the parathyroid autotransplantation and parathyroid inadvertent resection rates from 16% to 4% and 14% to 3%.[42]

Even though NIRAF can help identify parathyroid glands, its effectiveness for preventing permanent hypoparathyroidism has not been proven. In a systematic review of 13 articles, NIRAF and ICG in thyroidectomy compared with naked eye surgery found a reduction in the short-term (8%, 95% CI, 5%:11%) and medium-term (1%, 95% CI, 0%:4%) hypocalcemia rates compared with conventional surgery (15%; 95% CI, 9%:23% and 5%; 95% CI, 2%:9%).[43] No significant effect was observed for permanent hypocalcemia with an odds ratio of 0.42 (95% CI, 0:6689.29) and a risk difference of -0.0046 (95% CI, $-0.0124:0.0032$).[43] Another systematic review supports NIRAF for improving temporary hypocalcemia with no significant difference in the rate of permanent hypocalcemia.[44] Of note, Lu and colleagues found a significant difference in the rate of inadvertent resection of parathyroid glands in the NIRAF group (7.65%, 55/719) compared with naked eye surgery (14.39%, 132/917). Until larger multicenter trials are done, it is difficult to know whether reducing the rate of temporary hypocalcemia can, in turn, prevent permanent hypocalcemia given that a significant reduction was noted in an inadvertent parathyroid resection and autotransplantation.[42] This technology may be more useful in complicated thyroid surgery cases or revisions where scar tissue or lymph nodes can be misleading, and where early identification of these glands and their blood supply is essential. To justify the cost of the equipment, further research would need to demonstrate utility for preventing permanent hypocalcemia.

NIRAF alone without the use of contrast is limited in terms of the depth of detection.[45] For the probe-based technique, it needs to come into direct contact with the parathyroid gland, akin to how a recurrent nerve monitor would function. The addition of ICG contrast has been reported to improve the depth but by how much is not clear. One should be aware that false positive findings have been reported to occur with colloid thyroid nodules, brown fat, and cancer cells because they may have endogenous fluorophores,[46–49] and false-negative findings can occur in malignant disease due to the strong background fluorescence of the thyroid tissue in such cases.[50]

For transoral robotic thyroid surgery, intravenous injection with ICG is being used to help with the identification of parathyroid glands during CND where the inferior parathyroid glands are at the greatest risk.[51] Kim and colleagues, found a lower rate of transient hypocalcemia in 55 patients undergoing CND with transoral robotic thyroidectomy for papillary thyroid cancer in patients that used both autofluorescence and fluorescence imaging (18.5%) compared with the 55 patients in the control group (26.7%).[52] Although these differences were not statistically significant, the number of lymph nodes harvested was significantly greater for the fluorescence imaging group (7.0) compared with the control group (4.8; $P = .004$).[52]

For hyperparathyroidism, failed parathyroidectomies can occur in 5% to 10% of primary cases due to the inability to identify or localize the diseased parathyroid glands. This failure rate is higher in revision cases.[53,54] The NIRAF technology is a promising adjunct to the endocrine surgeon; however, further research for improving the quantification of the NIRAF differences between normal versus abnormal parathyroid glands found in familial, primary and secondary or tertiary hyperparathyroidism are needed. Different patterns of autofluorescence have been noted depending on the cause of hyperparathyroidism; however, the data are still limited.[55] Adenomas seem to exhibit a darker and more heterogenous NIRAF pattern compared with nonsecreting, suppressed glands.[56] Pathologic parathyroid glands may lose the ability to emit strong, homogenous autofluorescence but the evidence for this needs to be confirmed with larger trials.[55–61] Berber and colleagues reported in their cohort of 12 patients with tertiary hyperparathyroidism that their parathyroid glands exhibited similar intensity to those with classic primary hyperparathyroidism; however, the signal was more homogeneous.[55] Larger multi-institutional trials to better delineate the autofluorescence signal differences are required.

Thermal Ablation Techniques for Treating Thyroid and Parathyroid Disease

Thermal or chemical ablation represents another significant advancement in endocrine surgery for improving quality of life in patients with benign or low-risk thyroid disease. There has been considerable interest worldwide, particularly with radiofrequency ablation (RFA); however, other thermal techniques such as laser thermal ablation, microwave ablation (MA), and high-intensity focused ultrasound (HIFU) have also garnered popularity as well as evidence for their use (**Table 1**).[62,64–80] Each approach is slightly different; however, directed ablation techniques share the common theme that they can be performed in an outpatient setting, without a general anesthetic, removal of the gland, an incision, and often without thyroid function disruption making this an attractive option for patients who do not wish to have surgery. This represents a significant advancement in our era as a means for decreasing the burden of using expensive operative time, reducing the downtime associated with surgical recovery, and improving the overall quality of life in patients with benign or low-risk malignancy. With the recent publication of the North American guidelines for thermal ablation use, more centers are likely to adopt this technology.[62]

Benign Thyroid Nodules (Nonfunctioning)

The most robust evidence available is for the treatment of benign nodules with RFA or LA.[64–67,79] In a meta-analysis (24 studies where 12 examined RFA and 12 for LA), both modalities were effective in significantly reducing the size of the nodule, improving compressive symptoms as well as cosmetic concerns.[64] It has been well established that most treated nodules maintain volume reduction for 2 to 3 years, and in some studies up to 5 years.[68,70–72] A subgroup analysis shows that the outcome for thermal ablation (RFA and LA) is far greater when the nodules are less than 30 cc (which is equivalent to 30 cm^3, or a nodule size of 5 × 3 × 2 cm).[64]

Two important factors that determine the outcome is the size of the nodule and the amount of energy delivered to ablate the nodule.[81] If the nodule is large (>30 mL), less energy is dispersed throughout the nodule, and a greater amount of time needs to be dedicated to ablation. Other considerations which may improve the efficacy of RFA and LA is whether the nodule has a spongiform appearance as well as the presence of intranodular vascularity.[81] As long-term results emerge worldwide, patients will be offered more consistent projected outcomes. Currently, RFA demonstrates a mean 5-year volume reduction rate of 67% after one session[70] and a reduction rate of 50% to 60% with 3 to 6-year follow-up for LA.[71] Other studies have shown that 2 RFA sessions were needed for 20% of the patients.[69] During clinical follow-up, when the nodule shows significant shrinkage at the first visit after RFA or LA treatment, the volume is likely to be stable overtime compared with those nodules that have a decreased response rate within the first 6 months follow-up and are more prone to regrowth in 4 to 5 years.[64,65,68] Future studies may look to ways for improving the outcome of thermal ablation in large goiters where the results for thermal ablation are less effective. Because the technique and technology evolves, newer ways to achieve complete ablation in a single session will be addressed.

As more long-term data accumulates for the use of thermal ablation, ideal patient selection can be further delineated to determine which nodule characteristics are predictive of a long-term response rate. Negro and colleagues developed a machine learning model to reliably identify nodules that are likely to have a volume reduction rate of greater than 50% at 12 months after 1 RFA treatment session.[81] Using cumulative ultrasound characteristics from 6 institutions (407 cytologically benign thyroid nodules), AI achieved an 85% accuracy rate with a positive predictive value of 95% (CI: 0.92–0.98) and a negative predictive value of 95% (CI: 0.92–0.98). This type of algorithm may play a role in helping to guide patients with their decision-making whether surgical removal or thermal ablation will be more beneficial for sustained nodule reduction. Moreover, machine learning can help find consistent patterns in nodule characteristics that may predict better long-term results in larger nodules and can be a useful tool to help with patient counseling regarding the number of sessions needed to achieve symptom relief. We anticipate that AI will be incorporated into

Table 1
Summary of the advantages and disadvantages of minimally invasive techniques

Method		Advantages	Disadvantages
RFA	Frictional heat is generated when radiofrequency waves pass through electrode, and further conduction generated from the ablated area	Susceptible to the "heat sink effect" for a controlled ablative effect	Ablation may be affected by "heat sink effect" or the presence of calcifications, fluid or fibrosis in the nodule
LA	Light energy is delivered through optical fiber into the target tissue by an electrical current	Delivers less total energy, may be safer in critical locations	Delivers less total energy, maybe less effective for larger nodules
Microwave	Uses electrical magnetic field	Delivers more thermal energy in a shorter period of time Reduced treatment time for large nodules	Rapid heating that is less responsive to the "heat sink effect" Thermal spread is not impeded as with RFA
HIFU	Uses sound waves to create tissue vibrations that convert into frictional heat	Noninvasive and does not require probe insertion into the nodule	Challenge to deliver energy to a small area without injury to surrounding tissue
Ethanol	Chemical ablation; causes cellular dehydration and coagulation necrosis	Cheap, no expensive equipment needed Effective for small encapsulated cystic nodules	Can be unpredictable; leakage can occur outside the lesion Requires multiple treatments

Heat sink effect: Tumors with near-by vessels have a cooling effect and may lead to incomplete thermal ablation.

Adapted from Orloff LA, Noel JE, Stack Jr BC, Russell MD, Angelos P, Baek JH, et al. Radiofrequency ablation and related ultrasound-guided ablation technologies for treatment of benign and malignant thyroid disease: An international multidisciplinary consensus statement of the American Head and Neck Society Endocrine Surgery Section with the Asia Pacific Society of Thyroid Surgery, Associazione Medici Endocrinologi, British Association of Endocrine and Thyroid Surgeons, European Thyroid Association, Italian Society of Endocrine Surgery Units, Korean Society of Thyroid Radiology, Latin America Thyroid Society, and Thyroid Nodules Therapies Association. Head and Neck. 2021;1-28.

the workflow both prethermal and postthermal ablation as a means for predicting and recording objective follow-up.

Functioning Thyroid Nodules

The results for thermal ablation of autonomously functioning thyroid nodules (AFTN) have been somewhat inconsistent.[72,74] Larger trials have emerged showing that this approach is beneficial for reducing antithyroid medications but is more effective when smaller nodules are targeted. In a multicenter retrospective trial with 361 patients, nodule reduction was significant at all time points after thermal ablation, with a significant difference in the withdrawal of antithyroid medications at 2 months (32.5%), 6 months (38.9%), and 12 months (41.3%).[72] The size of the nodule played a major role as to whether medical therapy could be withdrawn, with the lowest rate (19%) for large nodules (>30 mL), compared with smaller sized (<10 mL) (74%) or medium-sized (49%) nodules. However, in a systematic review and meta-analysis of a similar cohort size (391 patients), nodule volume was not found to have a significant difference in thyroid stimulating hormone (TSH) normalization ($P = .54$) or volume reduction rate (VRR) ($P = .94$).[73] TSH normalization was achieved in 71.2% patients and volume reduction rate was 69.4% at a mean follow-up period of 12.8 months.

Future studies may focus on the technical aspects of thermal ablation for AFTN and on how to achieve TSH normalization with complete and confident vascular ablation with larger thyroid nodules.

Differentiated Thyroid Cancer

Due to the frequency of incidental detection of papillary thyroid microcarcinomas (PTMC), thermal ablation potentially represents a significant advancement in the treatment of patients with low-risk disease. However, patient selection is key when treating malignant thyroid disease with thermal ablation and involvement of a multidisciplinary team is essential. Thermal ablation is controversial for malignant disease but is considered as an alternative option once all traditional methods have been exhausted. Surgery still remains the treatment of choice for primary thyroid carcinoma, particularly for patients with aggressive histologic subtypes (such as tall cell variant, hobnail variant, columnar cell variant, diffuse sclerosing, or solid variant), evidence of metastatic lymphadenopathy, extrathyroidal extension, or for patients that are fit to undergo a general anesthetic.[62,82] Patients with multiple malignant nodules are also better served by surgery even if the nodules do not display extracapsular spread. Those nodules that sit close to the posterior thyroid capsule and abut the "danger triangle" run the risk of thermal spread to the RLN and are better served with surgery to ensure a clean dissection.[63]

Many of the international guidelines agree that minimally invasive techniques (thermal ablation) are best suited to patients with papillary thyroid microcarcinoma, similar to the indications for active surveillance, where the data is robust for efficacy and safety.[62,74,75] The data continues to rapidly evolve in this area, with long-term data showing a 98% to 100% complete disappearance of tumors up to 5-year follow-up after RFA treatment.[77,78]

Thermal ablation has the potential to be indispensable for treating locally recurrent thyroid cancer where the risk for reoperation is significant. In a systematic review of 18 articles (321 patients with 498 lymph node metastases), the volume reduction rate was 88.4% with a significant reduction in thyroglobulin measurements after thermal ablation ($P < .0001$).[80] When ablation was done for recurrent lymph nodes in the central compartment, the incidence of RLN injury was 6.23% (20/321), with temporary injury and complete recovery in 16 patients but permanent paralysis in 4 patients. This highlights the need to be cautious when approaching the central compartment: even though the technique is minimally invasive, there is potential risk to the nearby "danger triangle."

Parathyroid disease

Since 2010, studies have shown thermal ablation to be an alternative to surgery for primary hyperparathyroidism and less so for secondary hyperparathyroidism.[83–88] Surgical removal of a parathyroid adenoma is an effective method for normalizing calcium and PTH levels. However, some patients wish to avoid surgery or have medical comorbidities that render them unfit for a general anesthetic. In a study by Ha and colleagues, of the 11 patients treated with RFA for their primary hyperparathyroidism, 63.6% (7 patients) after RFA resulted in normalized levels of PTH, whereas 4 patients failed to reach biochemical normalization.[88] The studies examining the effects of RFA or ethanol are limited by a low enrollment of patients and duration of follow-up is up to 12 months compared with articles examining the effects of MA (up to 32 months).

Artificial Intelligence in Diagnostic Imaging

AI has emerged in many fields of medicine. Deep learning is being integrated into endocrinology as a means for improving the accuracy and diagnostic performance of ultrasound or sestamibi scans. AI is also being used as a way of rapidly triaging the increasing number of incidentally detected thyroid nodules to reduce the burden on health-care services. Specifically, several studies have compared AI with the interpretation by clinicians for determining whether a thyroid nodule requires biopsy.[89–92] The results for deep learning in thyroid imaging are promising and have been reported to show significant improvement in predicting malignancy over radiologists using the Thyroid Imaging, Reporting and Data System (TI-RADS) proposed by the American College of Radiology (ACR)[90] and/or matches the performance of radiologists.[91]

In a multicenter study (7 hospitals), Liang and colleagues found improved diagnostic accuracy when using an assisted deep-learning strategy (ThyNet) in the form of a video to mimic the live clinical setting during the evaluation of the thyroid. The combined ACR TI-RADS approach by radiologists with AI assistance (ThyNet) significantly improved the negative predictive value (93.2%) for benign nodules with an ACR TIRADS score of 3 to 6 points where decision-making for biopsy can be ambiguous. The positive predictive value for malignancy an ACR TIRADS score of 10 to 15 points was more than 95%.[89] Overall, the number of fine needle aspirations decreased from 61.9% to 35.2% using the ThyNet-assisted strategy while missed malignancy rates decreased from 18.9% to 17%. Such technology is not meant to replace human decision-making but rather enhance workflow where hospitals are overburdened with an increasing rate of incidental thyroid nodules.

Hyperparathyroidism is a wide spectrum of disease that includes primary hyperparathyroidism due to a hypersecreting parathyroid adenoma, parathyroid hyperplasia, and, more rarely, parathyroid carcinoma. AI is being explored as a means for improving preoperatively detection of abnormal parathyroid glands and can be used in conjunction with the preoperative workup or intraoperatively to help with the decision-making.[93–97]

Apostolopoulos and colleagues examined 632 parathyroid Tc-99m Sestamibi scans using an AI system called ParaNet to discriminate between patients with abnormal parathyroid glands (PG) and patients with normal PG in a cohort with primary hyperparathyroidism (607 patients), or refractory secondary or tertiary hyperparathyroidism due to renal disease.[93] These results are promising with a PPV of 98.76% and NPV of 91.57% using ParaNet. However, they may be artificially elevated due to the high number of patients with primary hyperparathyroidism, which may be easier to detect on imaging comparatively. Nonetheless, AI technology may assist with imaging acquisition and be embedded in the framework so a diagnosis can be achieved quickly.

Visual AI platforms are also being used to assist surgeons intraoperatively in the recognition of parathyroid glands by quantifying the signal of parathyroid autofluorescence. AI is being used to quantify and compare the autofluorescence signal of normal and abnormal parathyroid glands based on the notion that normal parathyroids exhibit a different pattern of autofluorescence.[98] Avci and colleagues found the sensitivity and positive predictive value of the model to be 89% for predicting normal and abnormal parathyroid glands.[99,100] Similarly, Akbulut and colleagues found that their algorithm for predicting normal versus abnormal glands was 95% accurate and 84% accurate in predicting subclasses of parathyroid pathologic conditions.[101]

SUMMARY

Endocrine surgery has made significant advances during the past several decades and continues to expand the surgical and nonsurgical techniques. Remote access thyroid and parathyroid surgery continues to push the boundaries of what can be done with the overall goal of improving the quality of patient care. Newer generation robotics are less cumbersome and easier to navigate in small cavities while attempting to recreate a sense of tactile feedback which is found in open surgery. The autofluorescence technology for identifying parathyroid glands is promising for reducing the rate of temporary and perhaps permanent hypoparathyroidism. Quantifying autofluorescence intraoperatively will likely become automated with AI whereby different emission patterns will help differentiate between pathologic and normal parathyroid glands. More long-term data will emerge for various types of thermal ablation confirming its oncological safety. Newer versions of the ablative techniques will incorporate recurrent nerve monitoring to ensure safety with higher temperatures. Future research will integrate AI to improve the workflow, safety, and diagnostic accuracy for preoperative assessment and intraoperative decision-making.

CLINICS CARE POINTS

- Newer generation robotics are being developed that are easier to navigate in small cavities, have a more ergonomic design, and incorporate tactile feedback.
- Augmented Reality has enabled visual imaging of the surrounding organs to help navigate nearby critical structures-Autofluorescence technology has shown to improve the temporary rate of hypocalcemia.
- Thermal ablation is oncologically safe for PTMC.
- Thermal ablation may be used for recurrent thyroid cancer that is not amenable to surgery for palliation.
- Artifical Intelligence is incorporated into the work flow of diagnostics in preoperative imaging, quantifying intraoperative autofluorescence signals, and for helping to differentiate normal from abnormal parathyroid glands.

DISCLOSURE

The authors have no financial disclosures to make. No funding was received. The authors have contributed to the writing, editing, and concept behind this study.

REFERENCES

1. Kim MJ, Nam KH, Lee SC, et al. Yonsei Experience of 5000 Gasless Transaxillary Robotic Thyroidectomies. World J Surgery 2018;42(2):393–401.
2. Kandil E, Hammad AY, Walvekar RR, et al. Robotic thyroidectomy versus nonrobotic approaches: A meta-analysis examining surgical outcomes. Surgical Innov 2016;23:317–25.
3. Lang BH, Wong CK, Tsang HS, et al. A systematic review and meta-analysis comparing surgically-related complications between robotic-assisted thyroidectomy and conventional open thyroidectomy. Ann Surg Oncol 2014;21·850–61.
4. Pan JH, Zhou H, Zhao XX, et al. Robotic thyroidectomy versus conventional open thyroidectomy for thyroid cancer: A systematic review and meta-analysis. Surg Endosc 2017;31:3985–4001.
5. Jackson NR, Yao L, Tufano RP, et al. Safety of robotic thyroidectomy approaches: Meta-analysis an systematic review. Head Neck 2014;36:137–43.
6. Wang YC, Liu K, Xiong JJ, et al. Robotic thyroidectomy versus conventional open thyroidectomy for differentiated thyroid cancer: Meta-analysis. J Laryngol Otol 2015l;129:558–67.
7. Yoon JH, Park CH, Chung WY. Gasless endoscopic thyroidectomy via an axillary approach: experience of 30 cases. Surg Laparosc Endosc Percutan Tech 2006;16(4):226–31.
8. Choe JH, Kim SW, Chung KW, et al. Endoscopic thyroidectomy using a new bilateral axillo-breast approach. World J Surg 2007;31(3):601–6.
9. Terris DJ, Singer MC, Seybt MW. Robotic facelift thyroidectomy: patient selection and technical considerations. Surg Laparosc Endosc Percutan Tech 2011;21(4):237–42.
10. Anuwong A. Transoral endoscopic thyroidectomy vestibular approach: a series in the first 60 human cases. World J Surg 2016;40(3):491–7.
11. Russell JO, Clark J, Noureldine SI, et al. Transoral thyroidectomy and parathyroidectomy – a North American series of robotic and endoscopic transoral approaches to the central neck. Oral Oncol 2017;71:75–80.
12. Richmon JD, Kim HY. Transoral robotic thyroidectomy (TORT): procedures and outcomes. Gland Surg 2017;6(3):285–9.
13. Anuwong A, Ketwong K, Jitpratoom P, et al. Safety and outcomes of the transoral endoscopic thyroidectomy vestibular approach. JAMA Surg 2018;153(1):21–7.
14. Russell JO, Noureldine SI, Al Khadem MG, et al. Transoral robotic thyroidectomy: a preclinical feasibility study using the da Vinci Xi platform. J Robot Surg 2017;11(3):341–6.
15. Dionigi G, Tufano RP, Russell J, et al. Transoral thyroidectomy: advantages and limitations. J Endocrinol Invest 2017;40(11):1259–63.
16. Razavi CR, Al Khadem MG, Fondong A, et al. Early outcomes in transoral vestibular thyroidectomy: Robotic versus endoscopic techniques. Head Neck 2018;40(10):2246–53.
17. Tamaki A, Rocco JW, Ozer E. The future of robotic surgery in otolaryngology – head and neck surgery. Oral Oncol 2020;101:104510.
18. Erkul E, Duvvuri U, Mehta D, et al. Transoral robotic surgery for the pediatric head and neck surgeries. Eur Arch Oto-Rhino-Laryngol 2017;274(3):1747–50.
19. Amirabdollahian F, Livatino S, Vahedi B, et al. Prevalence of haptic feedback in robot-mediated surgery: a systematic review of literature. Journal of Robotic Surgery 2017;12:11–25.

20. Abiri A, Juo YY, Tao A, et al. Artificial Palpation in Robotic Surgery using Haptic Feedback. Surg Endosc 2020;33(4):1252–9.
21. Razavi CR, Tanavde V, Shaear M, et al. Simulations and simulators in head and neck endocrine surgery. Ann Thyroid 2020;5:3.
22. Lee D, Kong HJ, Kim D, et al. Preliminary study on application of augmented reality visualization in robotic thyroid surgery. Annals of Surgical Treatment and Research 2018;95(6):297–302.
23. Lee D, Yu HW, Kim S, et al. Vision-based tracking system for augmented reality to localize recurrent laryngeal nerve during robotic thyroid surgery. Sc Rep 2020;10(1):8437.
24. Shuhaiber JH. Augmented Reality in Surgery. Arch Surg 2004;139:170–4.
25. Wang T, Wu Y, Xie Q, et al. Safety of central compartment neck dissection for transoral endoscopic thyroid surgery in papillary thyroid carcinoma. Jpn J Clin Oncol 2020;50(4):387–91.
26. Ahn JH, Yi JW. Transoral endoscopic thyroidectomy for thyroid carcinoma: outcomes and surgical completeness in 150 single – surgeon cases. Srg Endosc 2020;34(2):861–7.
27. Kim SY, Kim SM, Makay O, et al. Transoral endoscopic thyroidectomy using the vestibular approach with an endoscopic retractor in thyroid cancer: experience with the first 132 patients. Surg Endosc 2020;34(12):5414–20.
28. Kim JK, Lee CR, Kang SW, et al. Robotic transaxillary lateral neck dissection for thyroid cancer: learning experience from 500 cases. Surg Endosc 2022;36(4):2436–44.
29. Zhang Z, Sun B, Ouyang H, et al. Endoscopic Lateral Neck Dissection: A New Frontier in Endoscopic Thyroid Surgery. Front Endocrinol 2021;12:79684.
30. Christakis I, Constantinides VA, Tolley NS, et al. Parathyroid autotransplantation during thyroid surgery. World J Endocr Surg 2012;4(3):115–7.
31. Sakorafas G, Stafyla V, Bramis C, et al. Incidental Parathyroidectomy during Thyroid Surgery: An Underappreciated Complication of Thyroidectomy. World J Surg 2005;29:1539–43.
32. Duclos A, Peix JL, Colin C, CATHY Study Group. Influence of experience on performance of individual surgeons in thyroid surgery: prospective cross sectional multicenter study. BMJ 2012;344:d8041.
33. Di Marco AN, Palazzo FF. Near-infrared autofluorescence in thyroid and parathyroid surgery. Gland Surg 2020;9(Suppl 2):S136–46.
34. Croce AC, Bottiroli G. Autofluorescence spectroscopy and imaging: a tool for biomedical research and diagnosis. Eur J Histochem 2014;58(4):2461.
35. Tjahjono R, Nguyen K, Phung D, et al. Methods of identification of parathyroid glands in thyroid surgery: A literature review. ANZ J Surg 2021;91(9):1711–6.
36. Graves CE, Duh QY. Fluorescent technologies for intraoperative parathyroid identification. Ann Thyroid 2020;5(26):1–12.
37. Kim DH, Lee S, Jung J, et al. Near-infrared autofluorescence-based parathyroid glands identification in the thyroidectomy or parathyroidectomy: a systematic review and meta-analysis. Langenbeck's Arch Surg 2022;407(2):491–9.
38. Thomas G, Squires MH, Metcalf T, et al. Imaging or Fiber Probe-Based Approach? Assessing different methods to detect Near Infrared Autofluorescence for Intraoperative Parathyroid Identification. J Am Coll Surg 2019;229:596–608.e3.
39. Demarchi MS, Karenovics W, Bedat B, et al. Intraoperative autofluorescence and indocyanine green angiography for the detection and preservation of parathyroid glands. J Clin Med 2020;9:830.

40. Solórzano CC, Thomas G, Berber E, et al. Current state of intraoperative use of near infrared fluorescence for parathyroid identification and preservation. Surgery 2021;169(4):868–78.

41. Yin S, Pan B, Yang Z, et al. Combined use of Autofluorescence and Indocyanine Green Fluorescence Imaging in the Identification and Evaluation of Parathyroid Glands during Total Thyroidectomy: A Randomized Controlled Trial. Front Endocrinol 2022;13:897797.

42. Benmiloud F, Godiris-Petit G, Gras R, et al. Association of Autofluorescence-Based Detection of the Parathyroid Glands during Total Thyroidectomy with Postoperative Hypocalcemia Risk: Results of the PARAFLUO Multicenter Randomized Clinical Trial. JAMA Surg 2020;155(2):106–12.

43. Barbieri D, Indelicato P, Vinciguerra A, et al. Autofluorescence and Indocyanine Green in Thyroid Surgery: A Systematic Review and Meta-Analysis. Laryngoscope 2021;131(7):1683–92.

44. Lu W, Chen Q, Zhang P, et al. Near-Infrared Autofluorescence Imaging in Thyroid Surgery: A Systematic Review and Meta-Analysis. J Invest Surg 2022;35(9):1723–32.

45. Ladurner R, Al Arabi N, Guendogar U, et al. Near-infrared autofluorescence imaging to detect parathyroid glands in thyroid surgery. Ann R Coll Surg Engl 2018;100:33–6.

46. Zaidi N, Bucak E, Okoh A, et al. The utility of indocyanine green near infrared fluorescent imaging in the identification of parathyroid glands during surgery for primary hyperparathyroidism. J Surg Oncol 2016;113(7):771–4.

47. Silver Karcioglu AL, Triponez F, Solorzano CC, et al. Emerging Imaging Technologies for Parathyroid Gland Identification and Vascular Assessment in Thyroid Surgery. A Review from the American Head and Neck Society Endocrine Surgery Section. JAMA Otolaryngology – Head and Neck Surgery 2023. https://doi.org/10.1001/jamaoto.2022.4421.

48. De Leeuw F, Breuskin I, Abbaci M, et al. Intraoperative near-infrared imaging for parathyroid gland identification by auto-fluorescence: A feasibility study. World J Surg 2016;40:2131–8.

49. Papavramidis TS, Chorti A, Tzikos G, et al. The effect of intraoperative autofluorescence monitoring on unintentional parathyroid gland excision rates and postoperative PTH concentrations – a single-blind randomized-controlled trial. Endocrine 2021;72:546–52.

50. Idogawa H, Sakashita T, Homma A. A Novel study for fluorescence patterns of the parathyroid glands during surgery using a fluorescence spectroscopy system. Eur Arch Oto-Rhino-Laryngol 2020;277:1525–9.

51. Park JH, Lee J, Jung JH, et al. Intraoperative assessment of parathyroid perfusion using indocyanine green angiography in robotic thyroidectomy. Journal of Minimally Invasive Surgery 2022;25(3):112–5.

52. Kim WW, Choi JA, Lee J, et al. Fluorescence imaging-guided robotic thyroidectomy and central lymph node dissection. J Surg Res 2018;231:297–303.

53. Simental A, Ferris RL. Reoperative Parathyroidectomy. Otolaryngol Clin 2008;41(6):1269–74.

54. Cron DC, Kapeles SR, Andraska EA, et al. Predictors of operative failure in parathyroidectomy for primary hyperparathyroidism. Am J Surg 2017;214:509–14.

55. Berber E, Akbulut A, Avci S, et al. Comparison of Parathyroid Autofluorescence Signals in Different Types of Hyperparathyroidism. World J Surg 2022;46(4):807–12.

56. Kose E, Kahramangil B, Aydin H, et al. Heterogeneous and Low-Intensity Parathyroid Autofluorescence: Patterns Suggesting Hyperfunction at Parathyroid Exploration. Surgery 2019;165(2):431–7.

57. Squires MH, Shirley LA, Shen C, et al. Intraoperative autofluorescence parathyroid identification in patients with multiple endocrine neoplasia type I. JAMA Otolaryngol Head Neck Surg 2019;145:897–902.

58. Takeuchi M, Takashi T, Shodo R, et al. Comparison of autofluorescence with near-infrared fluorescence imaging between primary and secondary hyperparathyroidism. Laryngoscope 2021;131(6):E2097–104.

59. Idogawa H, Sakashita T, Homma A. A Novel study for fluorescence patterns of the parathyroid glands during surgery using a fluorescence spectroscopy system. Eur Arch Oto-Rhino-Laryngol 2020;277:1525–9.

60. Demarchi MS, Karenovics W, Bedat B, et al. Autofluorescence pattern of parathyroid adenomas. BJS Open 2021;5(1):zraa047.

61. Merrill AL, Sims SS, Dedhia PH, et al. Near-infrared Autofluorescence features of Parathyroid Carcinoma. Journal of the Endocrine Society 2022;6:1–5.

62. Orloff LA, Noel JE, Stack BC Jr, et al. Radiofrequency ablation and related ultrasound-guided ablation technologies for treatment of benign and malignant thyroid disease: An international multidisciplinary consensus statement of the American Head and Neck Society Endocrine Surgery Section with the Asia Pacific Society of Thyroid Surgery, Associazione Medici Endocrinologi, British Association of Endocrine and Thyroid Surgeons, European Thyroid Association, Italian Society of Endocrine Surgery Units, Korean Society of Thyroid Radiology, Latin American Thyroid Society, and Thyroid Nodules Therapies Association. Head Neck 2021;1–28.

63. Park HS, Baek JH, Choi YJ, et al. Innovative Techniques for Image-Guided Ablation of Benign Thyroid Nodules: Combined Ethanol and Radiofrequency Ablation. Korean J Radiol 2017;18(3):461–9.

64. Trimboli P, Castellana M, Sconfienza LM, et al. Efficacy of thermal ablation in benign non-functioning solid thyroid nodule: A systematic review and meta-analysis. Endocrine 2020;67(1):35–43.

65. Gharib H, Papini E, Garber JR, et al, AACE/ACE/AME Task Force on Thyroid Nodules. AACE/ACE/AME Task Force on Thyroid Nodules. American Association of Clinical Endocrinologists, American College of Endocrinology, And Associazione Medici Endocrinologi Medical Guidelines For Clinical Practice for the Diagnosis And Management of Thyroid Nodules – 2016 update. Endocr Pract 2016;22(5 Supple 1):622–39.

66. Kim JH, Baek JH, Lim HK, et al, Guideline Committee for the Korean Society of Thyroid Radiology KSThR and Korean Society of Radiology. Guideline Committee for the Korean Society of Thyroid Radiology (KSThR) and Korean Society of Radiology. 2017 Thyroid Radiofrequency Ablation Guideline: Korean Society of Thyroid Radiology. Korean J Radiol 2018;19(4):632–55.

67. Papini E, Pacella CM, Solbiati LA, et al. Minimally-invasive treatments for benign thyroid nodules: A Delphi-based consensus statement from the Italian minimally-invasive treatments of the thyroid (MITT) group. Int J Hyperthermia 2019;36(1):376–82.

68. Negro R, Greco G. Unfavorable outcomes in solid and spongiform thyroid nodules treated with laser ablation. A 5-year follow-up retrospective study. Endocr Meta Immune Disord Drug Targets 2019;19(7):1041–5.

69. Jung SL, Baek JH, Lee JH, et al. Efficacy and safety of Radiofrequency Ablation for Benign Thyroid Nodules: A Prospective Multicenter Study. Korean J Radiol 2018;19(1):167–74.
70. Deandrea M, Trimboli P, Garino F, et al. Long-Term Efficacy of a Single Session of RFA for Benign Thyroid Nodules: A Longitudinal 5-year Observational Study. J Clin Endocrinol Metab 2019;104(9):3751–6.
71. Papini E, Rago T, Gambelunghe G, et al. Long-term efficacy of ultrasound-guided laser ablation for benign solid thyroid nodules. Results of a three year multicenter prospective randomized trial. J Clin Endocrinol Metab 2014;99(10):3653–9.
72. Mauri G, Papini E, Bernardi S, et al. Image-guided thermal ablation in autonomously functioning thyroid nodules. A retrospective multicenter three-year follow-up study from the Italian Minimally Invasive Treatment of the Thyroid (MITT) Group. Eur Radiol 2022;32:1738–46.
73. Kim HJ, Cho SJ, Baek JH, et al. Efficacy and safety of thermal ablation for autonomously functioning thyroid nodules: a systematic review and meta-analysis. Eur Radiol 2021;31(2):605–15.
74. Mauri G, Hegedus L, Bandula S, et al. European Thyroid Association and Cardiovascular and Interventional Radiological Society of Europe 2021 Clinical Practice Guideline for the Use of Minimally Invasive Treatments in Malignant Thyroid Lesions. Eur Thyroid J 2021;10:185–97.
75. Kim JH, Baek JH, Lim HK, et al, Guideline Committee for the Korean Society of Thyroid Radiology KSThR and Korean Society of Radiology. 2017 Thyroid Radiofrequency Ablation Guideline: Korean Society of Thyroid Radiology. Thyroid 2018;19(4):632–55.
76. Xue JN, Teng DK, Wang H. Over than three-year follow-up results of thermal ablation for papillary thyroid carcinoma: A systematic review and meta-analysis. Front Endocrinol 2022;13:971038.
77. Cho SJ, Baek SM, Lim HK, et al. Long-Term Follow-Up results of Ultrasound-Guided Radiofrequency Ablation for Low-Risk Papillary Thyroid Microcarcinoma: More than 5-year Follow up for 84 tumors. Thyroid 2020;30(12):1745–51.
78. Cho SJ, Baek SM, Na DG, et al. Five-Year follow-up results of thermal ablation for low-risk papillary thyroid microcarcinomas: systematic review and meta-analysis. Eur Radiol 2021;31(9):6446–56.
79. Jasim S, Patel K, Randolph G, et al. American Association of Clinical Endocrinology Disease State Clinical Review: The Clinical Utility of Minimally Invasive Interventional Procedures in the Management of Benign and Malignant Thyroid Lesions. Endocr Pract 2022;28(4):433–48.
80. Zhang X, Ni T, Zhang W. Ultrasonography-Guided Thermal Ablation for Cervical Lymph Node Metastasis of Recurrent Papillary Thyroid Carcinoma: Is it Superior to Surgical Resection? Front Endocrinol 2022;13:907195.
81. Negro R, Rucco M, Creanza A, et al. Machine Learning Prediction of Radiofrequency Thermal Ablation Efficacy: A New Option to Optimize Thyroid Nodule Selection. Eur Thyroid J 2020;9:205–12.
82. Haugen BR, Alexander EK, Bible KC, et al. 2015 American Thyroid Association Management Guidelines for Adult Patients with Thyroid Nodules and Differentiated Thyroid Cancer. Thyroid 2016;26(1):1–133.
83. Fan BQ, He XW, Chen HH, et al. US-guided microwave ablation for primary hyperparathyroidism: a safety and efficacy study. Eur Radiol 2019;29:5607–16.
84. Korkusuz H, Wolf T, Grunwald F. Feasibility of bipolar radiofrequency ablation in patients with parathyroid adenoma: a first evaluation. Int J Hyperthermia 2018;34:639–43.

85. Liu F, Yu X, Liu Z, et al. Comparison of ultrasound-guided percutaneous microwave ablation and parathyroidectomy for primary hyperparathyroidism. Int J Hyperthermia 2019;36:835–40.

86. Kovatcheva R, Vladhow J, Stoinov J, et al. US-guided high-intensity focused ultrasound as a promising non-invasive method for treatment of primary hyperparathyroidism. Eur Radiol 2014;24:2052–8.

87. Andrioli M, Riganti F, Pacella CM, et al. Long-term effectiveness of ultrasound-guided laser ablation of hyperfunctioning parathyroid adenomas: present and future perspectives. AJR Am J Roetgenol 2012;199:1164–8.

88. Ha EJ, Baek JH, Baek SM. Minimally Invasive Treatment for Benign Parathyroid Lesions: Treatment Efficacy and Safety Based on Nodule Characteristics. Korean J Radiol 2020;21(12):1388–97.

89. Peng S, Liu Y, Lv W, et al. Deep learning-based artificial intelligence model to assist thyroid nodule diagnosis and management: a multicenter diagnostic study. Lancet Digital Health 2021;3(4):E250–9.

90. Liang J, Huan X, Hu H, et al. Predicting malignancy in thyroid nodules: radiomics score versus 2017 american college of radiology thyroid imaging, reporting and data system. Thyroid 2018;28:1024–33.

91. Buda M, Wildman-Tobriner B, Hoang JK, et al. Management of thyroid nodules seen on US images: deep learning may match performance of radiologist. Radiology 2019;292:695–701.

92. AIBx, Haertling T. Artificial intelligence model to risk stratify thyroid nodules. Thyroid 2020;30:878–84.

93. Apostolopoulos ID, Papthanasiou ND, Apostolopoulos DJ. A Deep Learning Methodology for the Detections of Abnormal Parathyroid Glands via Scintigraphy with 99mTc-Sestamibi. Diseases 2022;56:1–10.

94. Sandqvist P, Sundin A, Nilsson KL, et al. Primary hyperparathyroidism, a Machine Learning Approach to Idenitify Multiglandular Disease in Patients with a Single Adenoma Found at Preoperative Sestamibi-SPECT/CT. Eur J Endocrinol 2022;187:257–63.

95. Yoshida A, Ueda D, Higashiyama S, et al. Deep Learning-Based Detection of Parathyroid Adenoma by 99mTc-MIBI Scintigraphy in patients with Primary hyperthyroidism. Ann Nucl Med 2022;36:468–78.

96. Somnay YR, Craven M, Mc Coy KL, et al. Improving Diagnostic Recognition of Primary Hyperparathyroidism with Machine Learning. Surgery 2017;161:1113–21.

97. Imbus JR, Rande RW, Pitt SC, et al. Machine Learning to Identify Multigland Disease in Primary Hyperparathyroidism. J Surg Res 2017;219:173–9.

98. Wang Bo, Zheng J, Yu JF, et al. Development of Artificial Intelligence for Parathyroid Recognition During Endoscopic Thyroid Surgery. Laryngoscope 2022;132(12):2516–23.

99. Avci SN, Isiktas G, Ergun O, et al. A visual deep learning model to predict abnormal versus normal parathyroid glands using intraoperative autofluorescence signals. J of Surgical Oncology 2022;126(2):263–7.

100. Avci SN, Isiktas G, Berber E. A visual deep learning model to localize parathyroid-specific autofluorescence on Near-Infrared Imaging: Localization of Parathyroid Autofluorescence with Deep Learning. Ann Surg Oncol 2022;29:4248–52.

101. Akbulut S, Erten O, Kim YS, et al. Development of an algorithm for intraoperative autofluorescence assessment of parathyroid glands in primary hyperparathyroidism using artificial intelligence. Surgery 2021;170(2):454–61.

Moving?

Make sure your subscription moves with you!

To notify us of your new address, find your **Clinics Account Number** (located on your mailing label above your name), and contact customer service at:

Email: journalscustomerservice-usa@elsevier.com

800-654-2452 (subscribers in the U.S. & Canada)
314-447-8871 (subscribers outside of the U.S. & Canada)

Fax number: 314-447-8029

Elsevier Health Sciences Division
Subscription Customer Service
3251 Riverport Lane
Maryland Heights, MO 63043

*To ensure uninterrupted delivery of your subscription, please notify us at least 4 weeks in advance of move.

Printed and bound by CPI Group (UK) Ltd, Croydon, CR0 4YY

03/10/2024

01040471-0016